Nutrition-related health is important for cholangiocarcinoma patients. Eating the right kinds of foods before, during, and after cancer treatment can help you feel better and stay optimistic during the disruption that a cancer diagnosis brings. Even when things feel out of control, how you choose to fuel your body is something that you can control. Being mindful of what you consume will allow you to keep your body at a healthy weight, maintain strength and healthy body tissue, and decrease side effects both during and after treatment.

This nutrition guide has been written with you in mind. Building and sustaining a healthy body despite the invasion of cancer cells is important for your overall well-being. The information within the pages of this guide provides the foundation to improve your health as advised by experts and includes easy-to-make recipes.

This resource gives you the information you need to eat the right amount of protein and calories that are important for healing, fighting infection, and having enough energy throughout your cancer journey.

Good nutrition is a worthy goal for each of us. I hope this resource will assist and even enhance your quality of life as you navigate this pathway.

Stacie C. Lindsey
CEO & Founder
Cholangiocarcinoma Foundation

1

A
Special
Thanks...

2

This resource is brought to you by the
Cholangiocarcinoma Foundation and following sponsors:

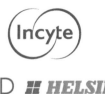

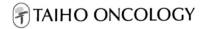

Special thanks to the authors:
Whitney Christie MS, RD, CSO, CNSC
Elizabeth Miracle MS, RD, CSO, CDN, CNSC
Stephanie Roit MS, RD, CDN, CSO
Katie Urban MS, RD, CDN

Design and graphics by
Albatross Book Co.

The Foundation would like to thank the Academy of
Nutrition and Dietetics and the Pancreatic Cancer Action
Network for their support and contributions.

Introduction

Cholangiocarcinoma is a rare form of cancer that affects the bile ducts of the liver. About 10,000 people in the United States develop bile duct cancer every year.

The bile ducts play an important role in normal **digestion** and nutrient **absorption** by moving fluid (**bile**) from the liver to the gallbladder to the small intestines, where it helps to digest the **fats** in food. The gallbladder functions to store bile produced by the liver and empties after a meal.

Cholangiocarcinoma may be **localized, locally advanced,** or **metastatic**. It may be **resectable** (able to treat surgically) or **unresectable**. **Surgery, chemotherapy, radiation, targeted therapies, immunotherapy,** and clinical trials are methods used to treat or control cholangiocarcinoma.

There are three types of cholangiocarcinoma: Intrahepatic, Perihilar (Hilar or Klatskin tumor), and Distal.

Liver

Gallbladder →

© Fran Miller 2017

Common Bile Duct →

Duodenum →

Intrahepatic: Develops in the small bile duct branches inside the liver.

Perihilar (Hilar or Klatskin): Develops where the left and right hepatic ducts have joined and are just leaving the liver. Also known as Klatskin tumors. These cancers are grouped with distal bile duct cancers as extrahepatic bile duct cancers

Distal: Found further down the bile duct, closer to the small intestine.

Each type of cholangiocarcinoma has differing treatment options. Because of the disease, treatments provided, and side effects associated with various forms of treatment, you may not feel like eating or may be curious about what you can eat to nourish your body. Nutrition plays a vital role in keeping your body properly functioning, optimizing your overall well-being, and helping you to feel your best.

Throughout this book, we hope to help make your journey a little easier by explaining the importance of nutrition throughout treatment and beyond. It offers nutritional guidance for various types of surgical procedures common to cholangiocarcinoma, and provides valuable tips for managing side effects that you may experience. In addition, recipes, meal plans, food charts, and resources are provided.

We work with individuals like you every day and are inspired by the strength you show as you courageously navigate this disease. We hope that this nutrition booklet will offer you some insight and helpful tips to nourish, strengthen and heal your body throughout your journey.

Pancreas

Nutrition and Cholangiocarcinoma

Choosing what to eat after a cancer diagnosis or while undergoing cancer treatment can be challenging or confusing.

Eating well can help decrease fatigue and the side effects of common treatments such as surgery, chemotherapy, and radiation.

Some cholangiocarcinoma treatments may cause a temporary or permanent change to how your body can process and absorb different nutrients. This booklet will provide general advice for managing common nutritional effects of cholangiocarcinoma. Working individually with a registered dietitian specializing in oncology is the best way to get tailored advice to meet your body's nutritional needs.

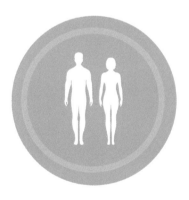

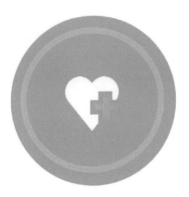

Role of the Registered Dietitian Nutritionist (RDN) in Your Care

Registered dietitians are the nutrition experts who can work with you to provide individualized dietary advice that considers your symptoms, preferences, and lifestyle to help you feel your best. A registered dietitian is trained in evidence-based practice to best understand the current research and how it applies to your treatment. They can provide credible information and answers to specific questions you may have about nutrition.

What is a Registered Dietitian?

A dietitian is someone who holds the title of Registered Dietitian (RD). A registered dietitian has completed an undergraduate and/or graduate degree in the study of nutrition and an internship that has been certified by the Academy of Nutrition and Dietetics. Upon completion of their studies, dietitians must pass a national registration exam administered by the Commission on Dietetic Registration. Some states require licensure; therefore, some dietitians may be both registered and licensed.

Anyone who has studied or has an interest in nutrition can call themselves a "nutritionist." The title "nutritionist" is not professionally regulated and does not signify an individual's level of knowledge, especially as it relates to cancer nutrition care.

All dietitians are nutritionists, but not every nutritionist is a dietitian.

Dietitians can provide credible and reliable nutritional information, especially for those undergoing cancer treatment.

How Can a Registered Dietitian Help?

A registered dietitian is a healthcare professional who can help those with cancer manage the side effects of treatment that affect the patient's ability to eat well. Registered dietitians can help with specific questions about the role of diet in cancer care and cancer prevention.

Since each patient is different, a dietitian can work with patients to meet their individual dietary needs.

02

Are There Dietitians Who Specialize in Cancer and Nutrition?

Yes! The Commission on Dietetic Registration offers a specialty certification in oncology nutrition. Dietitians must complete at least 2,000 hours of work in the oncology field and pass an examination in oncology nutrition to receive board certification. These dietitians have the additional credential "CSO" to indicate that they are a "Certified Specialist in Oncology" Nutrition.

The Oncology Nutrition Dietetic Practice Group (ON DPG) brings together dietitians across the country who work with patients seeking to either decrease their risk for cancer or eat well during and after cancer treatment. The ON DPG is a part of the Academy of Nutrition and Dietetics (AND), the world's largest group of food and nutrition professionals.

Where Can I Find A Registered Dietitian or Certified Specialist in Oncology Nutrition?

√ Ask the patient's oncologist for a recommendation

√ Contact a local hospital or cancer treatment center

√ Refer to the Oncology Nutrition Practice Group's website, oncologynutrition.org

√ Refer to the Academy of Nutrition and Dietetics website, eatright.org for more information and to search for a local dietitian

√ Visit the website for the Commission on Dietetic Registration, cdrnet.org for a list of Board Certified Specialists in Oncology Nutrition by state

NOTES

02

American Institute for Cancer Research (AICR)

The American Institute for Cancer Research regularly publishes and updates nutrition and exercise guidelines for Americans for cancer prevention and cancer survivors. Adopting these guidelines can help improve overall health.

1   Be a healthy weight. Keep your weight within a healthy range and avoid weight gain during adult life.

2   Eat a diet rich in whole grains, vegetables, fruit, and beans.

3   Be physically active as part of everyday life.

4   Limit consumption of fast foods and other processed foods that are high in fat, starches, or sugars.

5   Limit consumption of red and processed meat. Eat no more than 12-18 ounces per week of red meat such as beef, pork, or lamb. Eat little if any processed meat.

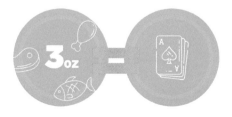

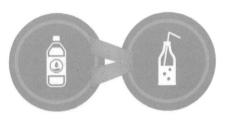

6   Limit consumption of sugar-sweetened drinks. Drink mostly water and unsweetened drinks.

7   Do not use supplements for cancer prevention. Aim to meet your nutritional needs through diet alone.

8   For mothers, breastfeed your baby, if you can.

9   Limit alcohol consumption.

10   After a cancer diagnosis, follow your doctor's recommendations.

For more information about the AICR nutritional guidelines, visit the American Institute for Cancer Research at AICR.org

General Nutrition Guidelines

The New American Plate

The New American Plate is a tool to help you build your meals to support your overall health and reduce your cancer risk. The New American Plate aims for a gradual transition from traditional meals that emphasize large portions of animal **protein** to a dietary pattern and plate that focuses on plant-based foods and whole grains. The New American Plate focuses on incorporating a variety of fruits, vegetables, whole grains, beans, or legumes.

These foods contain important **vitamins**, minerals, **fiber,** and phytochemicals that benefit health and can aid in cancer prevention.

√ The New American Plate suggests having fruits, vegetables, whole grains, beans, or legumes comprising ⅔ of the plate and ⅓ of the plate coming from animal proteins.

14

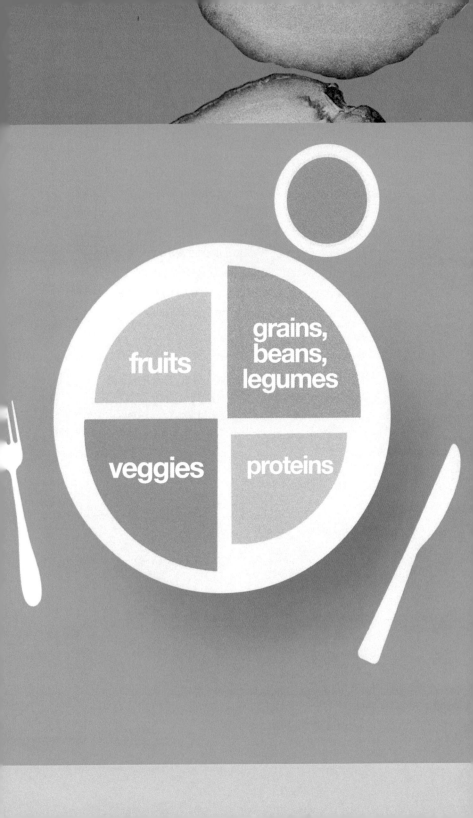

Goals of Nutrition Care
During Cancer Treatment

Nutrition care is an important aspect of your cancer care to help prevent or address malnutrition and cachexia (p 17), manage nutritional side effects of cancer treatments, and improve energy level and quality of life. Short-term goals of nutrition therapy may include increased calorie intake and symptom management, while long-term goals may include weight maintenance/gain/loss, increased muscle tone and strength, and decreased risk for chronic illness.

Because each person is unique,
goals will be individualized
and will likely change over
the course of your treatment.

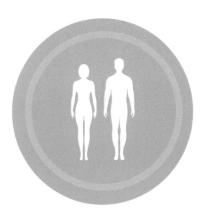

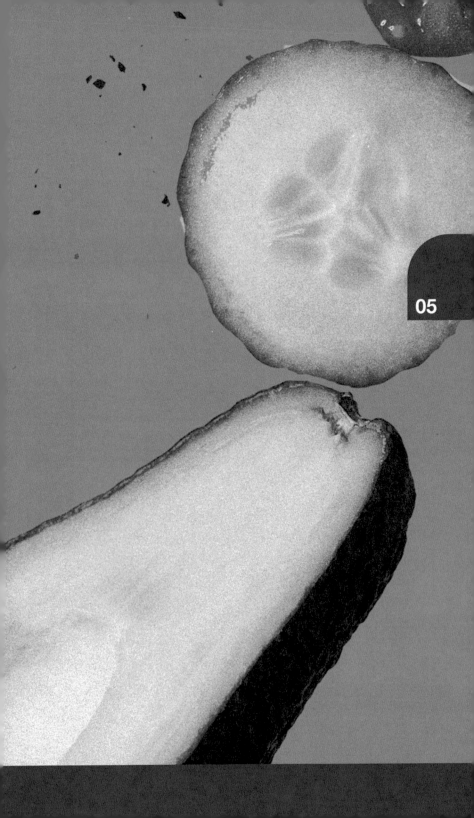

05

Malnutrition in the Setting of Cancer

Nutrition needs may change during cancer treatment, and it is important to ensure you get enough **calories**, **protein, fluids,** and **micronutrients** to stay healthy and tolerate treatment. Inadequate nutrition, referred to as malnutrition, can lead to weight loss, fatigue, and reduced quality of life during treatment. If you are not eating well, the common side effects of treatments may be more intense.

> If you're feeling nauseous, it helps to avoid an empty stomach. Snack on dry, salty foods such as pretzels or Saltines® to settle your stomach

Malnutrition is typically defined by multiple markers and can include decreased calorie intake, weight loss, loss of muscle mass or body fat, fluid accumulation, and reduced hand grip strength. The Academy of Nutrition and Dietetics and American Society for Parenteral and Enteral Nutrition (ASPEN) has outlined criteria to define malnutrition in the context of acute illness, chronic illness, or social/environmental circumstances that include these markers.

Malnutrition is particularly prevalent in patients who have been diagnosed with cancer due to increased nutrition needs, decreased oral intake due to side effects, and alterations to the absorption of nutrients. It can be mild, moderate, or severe in degree. It is important to discuss with your doctor and/or dietitian if you notice changes to these markers:

Markers to watch for:

- √ Weight loss
- √ How much you are eating if it is less than usual
- √ Loss of muscle mass or body fat
- √ Swelling in your legs, arms, or abdomen area
- √ Decreased hand grip strength

Weight loss that is unintentional over a quick timeframe is considered significant and may be a sign of malnutrition. The chart below outlines when weight loss is considered to be significant.

If you have lost weight, even if less than what is shown here, speak with your oncologist and/or dietitian.

Significant weight loss % and timeframe	Significant weight loss if you weigh:		
	125 lbs.	150 lbs.	200 lbs.
5% in 1 month	6 lbs	8 lbs	10 lbs
7.5% in 3 months	9 lbs	11 lbs	15 lbs
10% in 6 months	13 lbs	15 lbs	20 lbs
20% in 12 months	25 lbs	30 lbs	40 lbs

Research has shown that avoiding or treating malnutrition may help with:

- √ Better treatment outcomes

- √ Improved quality of life and reduced fatigue

- √ Reduced treatment toxicities and treatment delays/breaks

- √ Improved healing of wounds and immune response

Cachexia

Cachexia is the loss of both fat and muscle mass in the setting of inflammation. Typically, cachexia progresses through stages. Cachexia can affect appetite, energy levels for day-to-day activities, and tolerance to cancer treatments. It can increase your body's breakdown of muscle mass, worsening malnutrition and fatigue. Definitions of cachexia can vary but generally include these signs:

Signs of Cachexia

- √ Weight loss greater than 5% of body weight

- √ Greater than 2% weight loss with either BMI less than 20 kg/m2 <u>or</u> muscle loss

- √ Losing weight despite usual food and beverage intake

For the Caregivers

Caregivers are individuals helping someone with a cancer diagnosis and may involve helping with various day-to-day activities such as preparing meals and emotional support. Patients with cholangiocarcinoma may experience loss of appetite, nausea, and other digestive changes. Food preferences and tolerances may change quickly.

Encouraging small meals and having easy-to-eat snacks available is generally best.

If you are helping to prepare meals for someone undergoing treatment, the sections of this booklet on symptom management and recipes can provide helpful tips. You may also consider attending their appointment with a registered dietitian. Taking time to care for yourself is also important. The National Cancer Institute and the American Cancer Society provide additional information and resources for caregivers of loved ones. The Cholangiocarcinoma Foundation also provides support for caregivers of cholangiocarcinoma patients.

NOTES

_____

_____

_____

_____

_____

_____

_____

_____

_____

_____

_____

_____

_____

_____

Nutrition After
Duodenal Stent Placement

Nutrition is an important part of your *survivorship.* The following sections address nutrition-related concerns that may be encountered during or post-treatment.

If you have a blockage or obstruction of the **duodenum,** a part of your intestine, food is unable to pass through the area and be digested normally. This can cause nausea, vomiting, bloating, and loss of appetite. Your doctor may recommend a **duodenal stent** or a hollow tube placed in your intestine to open the blocked area and allow normal passage of food and liquids. It is important after stent placement to consume a diet that is soft, low in fiber, easy to chew and swallow to help prevent the stent from getting blocked or dislodged.

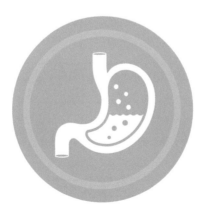

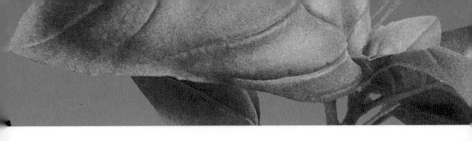

General Recommendations

- √ Try to have 5-6 small meals throughout the day instead of 2-3 larger meals.

- √ Sit upright when eating to allow gravity to help with your digestion. Avoid laying down for 30 minutes to 1 hour after eating.

- √ Limit drinking liquids with meals to avoid filling up quickly and to help with nausea. Try and consume any liquids 30 to 60 minutes before or after meals.

- √ Incorporate nutritional supplements between (not with) meals to increase calorie and protein intake.

- √ Limit high fiber foods immediately after stent placement. These include fresh fruit, vegetables, and whole grains.

- √ If you are prescribed medication to help with your intestinal **motility**, take it as directed by your physician.

- √ Note these are general guidelines. Foods allowed on this list may vary based on institution or healthcare providers.

Post-Stent Diet

	Recommended Foods	Foods *Not* Recommended
Fruits	Applesauce Bananas Cooked or canned fruits without skin or seeds (canned peaches, pears; baked apples without skin)	Dried fruit (raisins, prunes, mangos, dates) Fruit with skins or seeds (raspberry, blueberry, kiwi, strawberry, grapes) Pineapple Orange Fruit compotes
Vegetables	Cooked carrots Mashed potatoes, baked potatoes (no skin) Cooked, peeled, and de-seeded zucchini Pureed squash	Raw vegetables Celery Corn, peas Cauliflower, broccoli Potato skin Green leafy vegetables, salad

	Recommended Foods	Foods *Not* Recommended
Meats/Meat Substitutes	Tender, well-cooked poultry Fish Eggs Tofu Ground meats/meatloaf Finely chopped tuna, chicken, or egg salad (no celery, onion)	Tough or dry meats Hot dogs or sausage with casing Smoked, cured, or processed lunch meat Shellfish Beans Seeds Nuts and nut butter Protein bars
Milk and Dairy	Milk or non-dairy milk alternatives Plain Greek, regular or non-dairy yogurt Soft cheeses Cottage or ricotta cheese Cream cheese Whipped cream Sour cream	Milk or non-dairy milk alternatives mixed with nuts, seeds, fresh or dried fruit chunks, coconut Fruited yogurt

08

	Recommended Foods	Foods *Not* Recommended
Grains	Cooked cereals such as oatmeal, Cream of Wheat®, Farina® or grits Well-cooked white pasta White rice Pancakes or waffles moistened with syrup Dry cold cereal softened with milk or non-dairy milk alternative	Whole grain bread or bread with nuts, seeds, or raisins Whole grain pasta or pasta made from beans or lentils High fiber or bran cereals Brown or wild rice Quinoa, lentils Popcorn, chips, crackers, or pretzels
Desserts	Pudding, custard sherbet, sorbet, ice cream gelatin, popsicles	Desserts with nuts, seeds, coconut, and dried fruit

	Recommended Foods	Foods *Not* Recommended
Other Foods	Butter, margarine Ketchup Mayonnaise Dressings Soy sauce Oils: avocado, canola, olive	Fresh herbs Whole spices (fennel, red pepper flakes, celery, poppy, or sesame seeds) Jam or jelly with seeds or whole fruit pieces
Beverages	Water Milk or non-dairy milk alternatives 100% fruit juice Coffee, tea Broth Oral nutrition supplements	Fruit juices with pulp (orange, pineapple) Carbonated beverages

08

Nutrition After Surgery

Surgery can have a short- or long-term impact on your nutrition and digestion. Each patient has individualized nutritional needs after surgery. Therefore, it is important to consult with a registered dietitian or doctor before making any dietary changes. The doctor or registered dietitian can help create a diet plan that is right for you based on your unique medical history, treatment plan, and symptoms.

Cholecystectomy

The gallbladder stores and releases bile, which helps to digest fat in your foods. A **cholecystectomy** is a surgery performed that removes the gallbladder.

Low-Fat Diet

A diet low in fat is sometimes required after surgery to control symptoms of bloating, gas pain, diarrhea, and **malabsorption**. A low-fat diet limits fat in the diet to 40-50 grams per day (see sample menu below). **Fat** provides essential fatty acids that our bodies cannot make, helps absorb certain vitamins, and is a good source of calories. Fat can be found in meat, dairy products, added oils, dressings, or spreads. Eating and maintaining a good nutritional status after surgery can be challenging; thus, it is important to consult with a registered dietitian or doctor about symptoms you are experiencing before making any dietary changes.

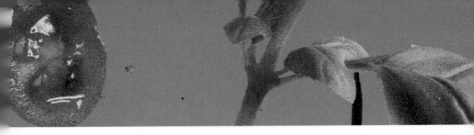

A low-fat diet may not solve all issues, so it is important to talk to your doctor or registered dietitian to help develop a meal plan that is right for you.

General Recommendations

√ Consume fats (as tolerated) and try to obtain from healthy sources such as olive oil, canola oil, peanut oil, nuts, seeds, and avocados.

√ Limit foods with more than 3 grams of fat per serving.

√ Avoid greasy and fried foods.

√ Bake, broil, steam, grill, boil, or roast meat, fish, and poultry versus frying or sautéing them in added fats.

√ Choose lean cuts of beef, pork, and other red meats (round or loin cuts).

√ Limit added fats such as butter, oils, margarine, mayonnaise, gravy, or dressings.

√ Remove chicken, turkey, and fish skins before consuming.

√ Choose non-fat, reduced, or low-fat milk (1% or 2% fat), yogurt and cheese products, or plant-based alternative dairy products.

Low-Fat Food and Snack Ideas

- √ Non-fat Greek yogurt with berries
- √ Rice cake with hummus and cucumber
- √ Egg white omelet with vegetables
- √ Popcorn (with olive oil and seasoning)
- √ Non-fat Greek yogurt dip with vegetables
- √ Turkey, low-fat cheese, and lettuce roll-ups
- √ Chicken, egg, or tuna salad with low-fat mayonnaise or hummus
- √ Non-fat cottage cheese or non-fat cream cheese with fruit and crackers
- √ Overnight oatmeal with low-fat dairy or dairy alternatives
- √ Low-fat pudding or gelatin
- √ Baked apple with cinnamon sugar
- √ Baked potato with salsa
- √ Non-fat frozen yogurt ice pops
- √ Frozen grapes

NOTES

09

Sample Meal Plan for Diet after Cholecystectomy Surgery

Provides: 1,755 Kcals, 45 g fat, 112 g protein

Breakfast

Oatmeal with almond milk, blueberries, and walnuts

1 cup oatmeal

2 tablespoon blueberries

1 cup almond milk

5 walnuts

Mid-Morning Snack

Egg Salad with cucumbers and tomato

1 hard-boiled egg, chopped

5 sliced raw cherry tomatoes

½ cup chopped cucumber

2 tablespoons chickpeas

1 tablespoon lemon juice

Salt and pepper

Lunch

Open-faced tuna melt

1 slice whole grain toast

½ cup canned tuna (in water)

2 slices tomato

2 ounces low-fat mozzarella cheese

Mid-Afternoon Snack
Greek yogurt with apples and cinnamon
6 ounces Greek yogurt
¼ apple, chopped
¼ teaspoon cinnamon
1 teaspoon honey

Dinner
Chicken Fajitas with a side of rice and corn salad
4 ounces grilled chicken breast
½ cup sliced red bell pepper
½ cup sliced onion
1 flour tortilla
¼ cup corn salad
½ cup brown rice

Evening Snack
**Graham crackers with low-fat cream cheese
and strawberries**
4 graham crackers
4 tablespoons low-fat cream cheese
4 strawberries, sliced

*Recipes for select meal items on page 112.

Liver Transplantation for Cholangiocarcinoma

Liver transplantation for cholangiocarcinoma may be considered for those with early-stage, unresectable intrahepatic or perihilar bile duct cancers. Liver **transplantation** involves removing the liver and bile duct, then transplanting a new liver when a suitable donor is identified. Nutrition is important after transplant to help you heal and to manage the short- and long-term side effects of anti-rejection medications.

General Recommendations

√ After your transplant, your appetite may be less than usual. Try and consume 5-6 small meals throughout the day instead of 2-3 larger meals.

√ Incorporate foods high in protein into your meals such as poultry, fish, beef, smooth nut butters, dairy products, and tofu. Try and consume protein portions of your meals first to help promote healing.

√ Incorporate nutritional supplement drinks between meals to increase calorie and protein intake.

√ Anti-rejection medications suppress your immune system and may make you more susceptible to foodborne illness. Follow food safety guidelines to reduce your risk. See below for a list of recommendations to minimize your risk of foodborne illness.

√ Some medications may increase your risk of **diabetes** or impact your blood sugar levels. If you have diabetes or issues with blood sugar control after surgery, eating well-balanced meals can help keep blood **glucose** levels close to normal.

Food Safety After Transplant

Food safety is an essential part of post-transplant nutrition care. You are at increased risk of foodborne illnesses as a result of the effect of post-transplant medications on your immune system. Foodborne illness can be severe requiring hospitalization.

Refer to the "Food Safety" Section on page 98 for further details regarding food safety and the steps you can take to keep yourself safe.

Other Nutritional Considerations

Medication Interactions

- ✓ **Immunosuppressive** medications such as **Cyclosporin** (Neoral®) or **Tacrolimus** (Prograf®) work to help your body accept the transplanted organ by suppressing your immune system. These medications interact with some foods, so it is important to avoid consuming them as part of your diet.

- ✓ These foods include grapefruit, starfruit, pomelo, Seville oranges, and pomegranates.

Changes in Appetite or Unintentional Weight Loss

Your appetite may be less than usual following your transplant, so it is important to include high-calorie/protein foods into your diet to support your recovery. Refer to High Calorie, High Protein page list (page 66) for further information and suggestions.

- √ Consume 5-6 small meals/day to improve your intake.

- √ Use high-calorie, high-protein nutritional supplements or homemade shakes.

Diarrhea

Diarrhea may occur as a side effect of your post-transplant medication regimen or because of an infection. Refer to the Diarrhea page (page 71) for further information and suggestions to help manage your symptoms.

- √ Limiting high fiber foods such as whole grains, fresh fruits, vegetables, whole nuts, and seeds may help prevent diarrhea.

- √ Incorporate foods like applesauce, bananas, white rice, white pasta, peanut butter, and cheese to help prevent diarrhea.

Fluid Retention

Medications used to suppress your immune system, such as **corticosteroids** (PredniSONE, Dexamethasone, MethylPREDNISone, Hydrocortisone), may cause your body to retain additional fluid after transplant. This can cause changes in your blood pressure. Making changes to your intake of sodium (salt) foods can help manage fluid retention symptoms.

- √ Limit sodium intake to less than 2,300 mg of sodium each day.

- √ Low sodium foods contain less than 140 mg of sodium per serving.

- √ Avoid processed, canned, or fast-food items. If using canned vegetables or beans/legumes, rinse under water prior to eating to reduce the sodium content.

- √ Limit added salt while cooking. Keep the saltshaker off the table during mealtimes. Try utilizing fresh or dried herbs or acids such as lemon juice or vinegar to add additional flavoring to foods.

High Blood Sugar (Hyperglycemia) and Diabetes

Medications used to suppress your immune system, such as Cyclosporin (Neoral®) or Tacrolimus (Prograf®), may also cause alterations in your blood sugar or **glucose** levels.

Dietary alterations to control portion sizes, limiting

simple sugars, and incorporating protein with **complex carbohydrates** can help control your blood sugar levels.

Your physician will monitor your blood sugar levels over time using a laboratory value called **hemoglobin A1C**, which measures your average blood sugar levels over a 2-3 month period.

√ Symptoms of high blood sugar include excessive thirst, hunger, urination, blurry vision, and dry mouth.

If your blood sugar levels do not improve, meet with your registered dietitian who can help you develop a meal plan.

High Potassium (Hyperkalemia)

09

Potassium is a mineral found in many foods that helps with heart function and muscle contraction. Normally, your kidneys regulate the amount of potassium in your body to prevent excess potassium from building up.

√ High blood potassium levels can cause muscle cramps, weakness, irregular heartbeat, and shortness of breath.

Transplant medications such as Cyclosporin (Neoral®), Tacrolimus (Prograf®), Bactrim™ and diuretic medications such as **Torsemide** (Demadex®), **Furosemide** (Lasix®) can affect levels of potassium in your blood.

If your potassium levels are out of the normal range (3.5-5.1 mmol/L), you may need to adjust your diet. Reach out to your transplant team and registered dietitian if you have specific questions about adjusting potassium in your diet.

Potassium Foods List

Low Potassium Foods
(<150 mg Potassium per serving)

- Apples
- Bean Sprouts
- Blueberries
- Cabbage
- Cranberries
- Cucumbers
- Dragon Fruit
- Grapes
- Grapefruits
- Guava
- Lemons
- Lettuce
- Limes
- Mushrooms
- Onions
- Peas (frozen, boiled)
- Pears
- Pineapples
- Turnips
- Watermelon
- Zucchini

Medium Potassium Foods
(200-350 mg Potassium per serving)

- Asparagus
- Cherries
- Chinese cabbage
- Cauliflower
- Carrots
- Celery
- Corn
- Dried Peas
- Leeks
- Lentils
- Okra
- Snow Peas
- Peaches
- Papaya
- Plums
- Pumpkin
- Raspberries
- Strawberries
- Tomatoes (raw, canned)

High Potassium Foods
(350 mg Potassium per serving)

- Apricots
- Artichokes
- Bananas
- Beet greens
- Broccoli (cooked)
- Brussels sprouts
- Cantaloupe
- Dates, figs, dried fruit
- Dried beans
- Kale
- Kiwi
- Honeydew
- Mango
- Mustard greens
- Nectarines
- Orange/orange juice
- Pomegranates
- Plantains
- Prunes/prune juice
- Salt substitutes
- Seaweed
- Spinach
- Starfruit
- Sweet potato
- Tomato juice
- Whole grains
- Winter squash
- Yams
- Yucca

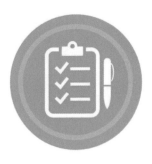

Whipple Surgery (Pancreaticoduodenectomy)

The **pancreas** helps with digestion by producing enzymes that help break down fats, proteins, and carbohydrates and producing bicarbonate, which helps neutralize stomach acid. The pancreas also produces insulin and glucagon, which help your body regulate and maintain blood sugar levels.

The Whipple surgery (Pancreaticoduodenectomy) involves the removal of the head of the pancreas, duodenum or part of the small intestine, the gallbladder, and sometimes part of the stomach. Eating and maintaining a good nutritional status after surgery can be challenging; thus, it is important to consult with a registered dietitian or doctor about symptoms you are experiencing before making any dietary changes and develop a meal plan that is right for you.

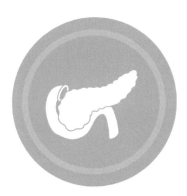

General Recommendations

- √ After surgery, your appetite may be less than usual. Try and consume 5-6 small meals throughout the day.

- √ Limit drinking liquids with meals to avoid getting full quickly and helping with nausea. Try and consume liquids 30 to 60 minutes before or after meals.

- √ Consume fat-containing foods as tolerated after surgery. Avoid greasy or fried foods. Refer to the Low-Fat Diet (page 26) section for further information.

- √ Incorporate foods high in protein into your meals such as poultry, fish, beef, smooth nut butters, dairy products, and tofu. Try and consume protein first to help promote healing.

- √ Incorporate nutritional supplement drinks between meals to increase calorie and protein intake. Talk to your registered dietitian or doctor about what supplement is right for you. Examples of available supplements can be found on page 102.

- √ Limit high-fiber foods immediately after surgery to help with digestion. These include fresh fruit, vegetables, and whole grains. Foods to avoid include broccoli, brussels sprouts, green leafy vegetables, cauliflower, corn, beans, and whole-wheat products.

- √ The pancreas produces insulin, a hormone that helps your body use glucose (sugar) in your blood. If you have diabetes or issues with blood sugar control after surgery, eating well-balanced meals can help keep blood glucose levels as close to normal.

09

- Limit consumption of simple sugars to help control both blood sugar levels and prevent dumping syndrome. **Dumping syndrome** is the rapid emptying of the stomach shortly after eating. It may be characterized by flushed skin, weakness, dizziness, abdominal pain, nausea, vomiting, and/or diarrhea.

- If prescribed **pancreatic enzymes**, take as instructed. Monitor your weight and stools for evidence you may not be absorbing fat well after surgery. Signs that you may not be absorbing fat include greasy, floating, foul-smelling, and light yellow or orange-colored stools. Talk to your doctor or registered dietitian if these symptoms are new to you or worsen.

Low-Fiber Diet

A low-fiber diet limits the amount of **fiber** you consume so your body can digest food more easily. This is important after surgery to facilitate healing and reduce inflammation. The low-fiber diet provides less than 13 grams of fiber each day. Low-fiber foods contain less than 3 grams of fiber per serving. Below are examples of foods you can eat to follow a low-fiber diet after your **Whipple surgery**. Note these are general guidelines. Foods allowed on this diet or recommended diet duration may vary based on institution or healthcare providers. Most patients are able to gradually reincorporate fiber into their diet.

09

Low-Fiber Diet

	Recommended Foods	Foods *Not* Recommended
Fruits	Applesauce Bananas Cooked or canned fruits without skin or seeds (canned peaches, pears; baked apples without skin)	Dried fruit (raisins, prunes, mangos, dates) Fruit with skins or seeds (raspberry, blueberry, kiwi, strawberry, grapes) Pineapple Orange Fruit compotes
Vegetables	Cooked carrots Cooked green beans Cooked, peeled, and de-seeded zucchini Mashed potato or baked potato with skin removed Pureed Squash Marinara Tomato Sauce	Celery, Corn, Peas Onion Green Leafy Vegetables (spinach, collard greens, kale) Broccoli, Cauliflower, Brussels Sprouts Cabbage Mushroom Peppers Tomatoes, chunky tomato sauces with skins/seeds

	Recommended Foods	Foods *Not* Recommended
Meats/Meat Substitutes	Tender, well-cooked, skinless poultry, beef, pork Fish or Shellfish Eggs Tofu, Seitan Ground meats/meatloaf Tuna or chicken salad (no celery, onion) Smooth nut butters (almond, peanut)	Tough or Dry cuts of meat Hot dogs or sausage with casing Beans Seeds Nuts or chunky nut butters
Milk and Dairy	Milk or non-dairy milk alternatives Plain Greek, regular or non-dairy yogurt Cheese Cottage Cheese or Ricotta Cheese Sour Cream Whipped Cream	Milk or non-dairy milk alternatives mixed with nuts, seeds, fruit chunks, or coconut Fruited yogurt

	Recommended Foods	Foods *Not* Recommended
Grains	Cooked cereals such as Cream of Wheat®, Farina®, Grits Cold Cereal such as Rice Chex®, Corn Flakes, Rice Krispies®, Cheerios™ White flour pasta, bread, rice White flour or finely ground corn tortilla White crackers without seeds (Saltines®, Ritz®) Pancakes or waffles Pretzels	Whole grain bread or bread with nuts, seeds, or raisins Whole grain pasta or pasta made from beans or lentils Whole grain tortillas High fiber or bran cold cereals Oatmeal Brown or wild rice Quinoa, lentils Popcorn
Desserts	Pudding, Custard Sherbet, Sorbet, Ice Cream, Frozen Yogurt Gelatin Lemon Drop Candy Popsicles Pound Cake	Desserts with nuts, seeds, coconut, or dried fruit

	Recommended Foods	Foods *Not* Recommended
Other Foods	Butter, margarine Ketchup Mayonnaise Soy sauce Dressings Oils: avocado, canola, olive	Fresh Herbs Whole Spices (fennel, red pepper flakes, celery, poppy, or sesame seeds) Jam or jelly with seeds or whole fruit pieces
Beverages	Water Milk or non-dairy milk alternatives 100% fruit juice (½ cup diluted 1:1 with water) Coffee, Tea Broth Flat carbonated beverages Oral Nutrition Supplements	Fruit juices with pulp (orange, pineapple) Carbonated beverages

09

Nutrition Following Whipple Surgery: Low-Fiber Snack/Small Meal Ideas

After surgery, you may fill up more quickly. It is recommended to have 5-6 smaller meals throughout the day. The following are snack or small meal ideas that you can include in your meal plan following surgery to help you get adequate calories and protein to facilitate healing and minimize symptoms you may be experiencing.

- ✓ White bread with smooth peanut or almond butter, banana, and honey drizzle.

- ✓ Smoothie (option to include Greek or plain yogurt, fresh fruit such as bananas, cantaloupe, honeydew, protein powder, smooth nut butters).

- ✓ Cottage cheese with cantaloupe.

- ✓ Cold cereal with milk or non-dairy milk alternative.

- ✓ Ricotta cheese or cream cheese with honey on white bread.

- ✓ English muffin pizza with mozzarella cheese and marinara tomato sauce.

- ✓ Hard-boiled or scrambled eggs.

- ✓ Tuna, chicken, or egg salad (no celery, onion) on white bread or white, seedless crackers.

- ✓ Mozzarella or cheddar cheese stick.

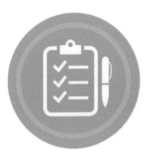

- Banana (option to add: smooth peanut or almond butter or dip in yogurt or chocolate and then freeze on a baking sheet).

- White flour cheese quesadilla (add chicken, tofu, or beef for additional protein, sour cream for additional calories).

- Mashed avocado on white, seedless crackers (option to drizzle with olive oil to add additional calories).

- Applesauce or fruit squeeze packs (Gogo Squeeze™).

- Plain Greek, regular or non-dairy yogurt (add canned peaches, sliced banana, 1 tablespoon of smooth peanut or almond butter).

- Pudding, ice cream, frozen yogurt, or gelatin.

- Graham crackers with smooth peanut or almond butter.

Sample Low-Fiber Meal Plan for After Whipple Surgery

Provides 1,766 calories, 80 g fat, 68 g protein, 13 g fiber

Breakfast

Greek yogurt with cantaloupe and cereal

1 cup Greek yogurt

2 tablespoons crispy cereal

½ cup cubed cantaloupe

Mid-Morning Snack

Smooth peanut butter, banana, honey on white toast

1 slice of white toast

2 tablespoons peanut butter

1 banana

1 teaspoon honey

Lunch

Creamy, pureed carrot ginger soup

1 cup carrot ginger soup

2 ounces coconut milk

Mid-Afternoon Snack

Egg Salad with crackers

2 hard-boiled eggs

2 tablespoons mayonnaise

5 Saltine™ crackers

Dinner

Lemon Orzo with shredded chicken and parmesan

1 cup orzo

½ cup shredded chicken breast

1 ounce shredded parmesan

1 tablespoon lemon juice

1 teaspoon chopped parsley

Salt and pepper

09

Evening Snack

Vanilla pudding with canned peaches

1 vanilla pudding

½ cup canned peaches

½ teaspoon cinnamon

*Recipes for select meal items on page 112.

Nutrition Support

Tube feeding (Enteral Nutrition) or IV Nutrition (Parenteral Nutrition)

During treatment, there may be times when your diet cannot meet nutritional goals due to surgery, side effects of chemotherapy, or the cancer itself. The following section reviews nutrition support methods that may be used short- or long-term during treatment to help you achieve adequate nutrition. Your physician or registered dietitian does not routinely recommend alternative nutrition methods but is chosen carefully based on your individualized survivorship plan and treatment goals.

Enteral Nutrition (EN):

If needed, during treatment your physician may recommend a feeding tube to help you get adequate nutrition. **Enteral nutrition** provides nutrition directly into your gastrointestinal tract bypassing your mouth. Your physician may consider a feeding tube if you are unable to get enough nutrition by mouth, based on side effects of chemotherapy, you have a blockage, or before/at the time of your surgery. A tube may be placed through your nose into your stomach (**nasogastric tube**), directly through your abdominal wall (**gastrostomy tube**), or inserted through the abdomen into the small intestine, bypassing the stomach (**jejunostomy tube**). Feeding tubes can be used at home or in the hospital setting to help optimize nutrition based upon your nutrition requirements, medical history, schedule, and needs.

A specialized liquid nutrition formula is used with your feeding tube to provide calories, protein, vitamins/minerals, and fluids. A registered dietitian will choose a formula that is right for your individualized nutritional needs. If needed, pancreatic enzymes can be used in a cartridge form using a product called **RELiZORB™** to help you digest and absorb your food. Over time, the nutrition formula provided through the feeding tube can be adjusted or discontinued entirely based on how you are eating. It is important to consult with a registered dietitian or doctor before making any changes to your prescribed liquid nutrition regimen.

Parenteral Nutrition (PN)

Parenteral nutrition is a form of intravenous (IV) nutrition that can supply nutrition through carbohydrates (dextrose), protein (amino acid), fat (lipids), vitamins, minerals, and trace elements. It is only used if you are unable to eat by mouth or receive enteral nutrition - typically when there is a blockage of the digestive tract, malabsorption, severe vomiting or diarrhea, **ileus**, or if prolonged bowel rest is required after surgery. Parenteral nutrition is provided through an IV inserted peripherally into a small vein (**peripheral line**) or centrally into a larger vein (**central line**). If started on PN, a physician and your registered dietitian will closely monitor your laboratory values, weight, and ability to transition back to an oral diet or enteral nutrition support. It is not routinely recommended during treatment.

oley.org/

The Oley Foundation is an excellent resource for individuals receiving tube feeding or intravenous nutrition. Adjusting to these forms of nutrition can take some time for both the patient and caregivers. Resources, support groups, and additional information can be found on their webpage.

Malabsorption and Pancreatic Enzymes

Exocrine Pancreatic Insufficiency (EPI)

A pancreas that functions normally produces **pancreatic enzymes,** which help your body break down the fat, protein, and carbohydrates in foods. These enzymes empty into the duodenum and aid in digestion. When you eat, varying levels of pancreatic enzymes are secreted based on the fat content and volume of the meal ingested. When your pancreas does not produce enough enzymes or has a blockage, your body may not be able to absorb fat as it normally would. This is called **exocrine pancreatic insufficiency** (EPI). It can result in fat **malabsorption** which can cause poor absorption of nutrients and can lead to malnutrition.

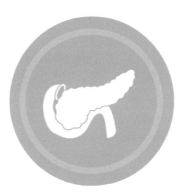

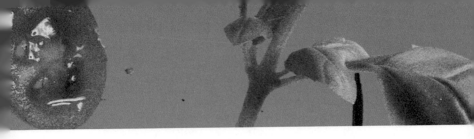

Causes of Malabsorption

Insufficient pancreatic enzyme production may be related to cancer itself or treatments for the cancer. Certain conditions can also disrupt the production or movement of pancreatic enzymes. In cholangiocarcinoma, EPI may be caused by:

- √ Whipple surgery (Pancreaticoduodenectomy)
- √ Blockage or narrowing of the pancreatic or biliary duct (the tubes that carry pancreatic enzymes or bile)
- √ **Distal Pancreatectomy**
- √ Tumors with pancreatic or small intestine involvement
- √ Some medical treatments (such as chemotherapy, radiation to the bowel, and surgery of the pancreas, stomach, or duodenum)
- √ Pancreatitis

Signs and Symptoms

Signs and symptoms of EPI or that you may not be digesting fat in your diet may include the following:

- √ Inability to gain weight
- √ Unintentional weight loss

- √ Fatigue

- √ Bloating or abdominal discomfort, particularly after meals

- √ Cramping or pain after meals

- √ Indigestion or burping

- √ Particles of undigested food in the toilet after bowel movements

- √ Bowel movements that are light in color (yellow, tan, clay-colored, or white)

- √ Foul-smelling bowel movements or gas

- √ Frequent, large, oily floating stools (**Steatorrhea** – typically does not occur until EPI is advanced)

Avoiding high-fat foods if you have one or more of the above symptoms is common; however, it may not always be right for you.

Patients with these symptoms should discuss with their medical team whether **pancreatic enzyme replacement therapy (PERT)** or making changes in their diet is beneficial for them.

Treatment

Pancreatic enzymes are used to treat EPI. Enzymes are available in pill, powder, or cartridge form. Pancreatic enzymes contain **lipase, protease,** and **amylase** to help facilitate the digestion of fats, proteins, and carbohydrates in the diet. They mimic what your pancreas would normally do.

It is important to take prescribed enzymes with meals and snacks. Pancreatic enzymes are taken at the smallest recommended dose and may be increased based on digestive symptoms, degree of steatorrhea (fatty stools), and the meal's fat content. Adequate enzyme dosing is needed to optimize pancreatic enzyme replacement therapy and improve symptoms of enzyme insufficiency.

There are six prescription pancreatic enzymes available: Creon®, Pancreaze®, Pertzye®, Ultresa®, Viokace®, and ZenPep®. Some individuals have more success with one enzyme brand. Insurance coverage for pancreatic enzymes can differ. Speak to your physician or registered dietitian about what enzyme product is right for you.

Tips for Taking Pancreatic Enzymes

√ Start with the smallest dose recommended. If you still have symptoms after eating, speak to your medical team as your dose may need to be increased.

√ Take your enzymes at the beginning of a meal or snack with the first bite of food. Pancreatic enzymes are effective for 45-60 minutes after they are taken.

11

- If taking more than one enzyme, take some at the beginning of your meal and the rest at various times throughout your meal.

- If you take multiple enzymes and struggle to take the number of enzymes recommended, ask your doctor, pharmacist, or registered dietitian about options to take fewer enzymes (such as switching to the highest strength offered).

- Pancreatic enzymes do not work well if taken at the end of the meal.

- Half of the prescribed dose is typically taken with snacks.

- You do not need to take pancreatic enzymes with fat-free foods or drinks.

- If having difficulty swallowing your enzymes, open the enzyme capsule and put powder on a spoonful of soft food such as applesauce, pureed bananas, or pears that can be easily swallowed. Before swallowing, do not mix enzyme spheres with milk, custard, ice cream, or other dairy products, as lactose may break down the enteric coating on the beads.

- Pancreatic enzymes do not work as well when taken with iron supplements, magnesium, or calcium-containing antacids.

Side Effects

When taken properly, pancreatic enzymes can help with digestion, weight gain, and quality of life by improving uncomfortable symptoms associated with EPI. Side effects of pancreatic enzymes can be similar to signs of pancreatic insufficiencies, such as nausea, abdominal cramps, or diarrhea. Taking too many enzymes may cause constipation. Speak with your doctor if you feel that your pancreatic enzymes are not working for you. You may benefit from a change in enzymes or your dosage.

Pancreatic Enzymes and Enteral Nutrition (Tube Feeding)

11

If you are receiving continuous enteral nutrition or nutrition through a feeding tube using a tube feeding pump and are experiencing symptoms of EPI, there is a cartridge that contains pancreatic enzymes called **RELiZORB™** available to help digest and absorb your tube feeding. The enzyme cartridge connects to the tubing, and the tube feeding formula flows through the cartridge. During this process, **lipase** in the enzyme cartridge breaks down fat in the formula allowing for improved fat absorption.

One to two enzyme cartridges can be used for up to 1000ml of formula in 24 hours. Tube feeding formulas containing

insoluble fibers are not compatible with RELiZORB™. Your tube feed rate should not exceed 120ml/hr. Your registered dietitian will work to select the right formula for you. For further information regarding tube feeding, please refer to the Nutrition Support section (page 52).

Financial Considerations

Similar to many prescription drugs, insurance coverage varies for pancreatic enzymes. Some insurance companies have a preferred brand that may lower copay costs. Most Medicare coverage drug plans have a "donut hole" or a temporary limit on what the drug plan will cover.

 If you are struggling with the cost of enzymes:

- √ Check with your insurance company to see if one brand is preferred over another.

- √ You may be eligible for Patient Assistance Programs offered by various pancreatic enzyme companies- visit the pancreatic enzyme manufacturer's website or visit NeedyMeds.org.

- √ If you are on Social Security, apply for the Extra Help plan.

- √ Contact your medical team for additional suggestions/resources. Ask if a financial counselor, nurse navigator, or social worker is available.

Other Considerations

Pancreatic enzymes are made from the pancreas of pigs. Individuals with allergies, ethical, or religious preferences related to **porcine,** or pig products should speak with their medical team to find an appropriate enzyme product for them.

Talk with your medical team if you continue to experience symptoms of fat malabsorption or unintentional weight loss. This may indicate that your pancreatic enzyme dose needs to be adjusted. Pancreatic enzyme tolerance and doses may need adjusting over time.

NOTES

_____

_____

_____

_____

_____

_____

_____

_____

Nutritional Management of Side Effects of Cancer Treatment

There are a variety of treatment options that are determined by your medical team for cholangiocarcinoma. With treatments often come side effects. These side effects can vary depending on the type of treatment received. For example, conventional radiation side effects are often "site-specific." With cholangiocarcinoma, radiation may be done to the liver or pancreas and may cause nausea/vomiting, fatigue, diarrhea, and/or loss of appetite. Chemotherapies (or immunotherapies) are another form of treatment and have common side effects known to the drugs used.

Please refer to the specific sections for nutrition-related side-effect management techniques that may help improve common problems associated with a variety of treatment types. Be proactive and ask your medical team to learn more about side effects commonly associated with specific treatments you are receiving. A registered dietitian may also be available to help provide more individualized nutrition counseling and resources.

Poor Appetite (Anorexia):

Appetite loss or decreased motivation to eat is common during cancer treatment. Nutrition plays a key role during treatment, so it is important to find a plan to manage appetite loss that works for you.

Tips to Manage Poor Appetite

√ Consume small frequent meals throughout the day; for example, consume 5-6 small meals rather than 3 larger meals.

√ Eat the most when you are feeling your best.

√ Eat by the clock versus diminished hunger cues. Schedule eating times with reminders on your phone using a timer or alarm.

√ Try having breakfast foods at other times of the day to increase variety.

12

√ Save meal leftovers for snacks at other times of the day. Keep easy to prepare meals on hand when cooking is tiring.

√ Incorporate full-fat dairy products (whole milk, yogurt, cheese) to increase the calorie content of meals and snacks, if able to tolerate.

√ Add avocado or extra condiments such as butter and/or olive or coconut oil to foods to increase the calorie content of meals and snacks.

√ Add nuts, nut butters, coconut, or dried fruit to snacks to increase the calorie content.

- ✓ Engage in light physical activity as allowed to stimulate appetite.

- ✓ Eat during an activity or with family and friends.

- ✓ Your physician may also prescribe medications to help stimulate your appetite, take as directed to help improve your intake level during treatment.

- ✓ Be sure to address with your doctor or registered dietitian any side effects such as nausea or pain that might be affecting your appetite.

Strategies to Increase Calories and Protein

It is important to consume enough calories and protein throughout the day during your cancer treatment to maintain strength, energy, and weight. Some tips on adding calories and protein may not seem like the healthiest choice; however, when your appetite is decreased, and side effects are inhibiting your meeting your nutrition goals, it may be beneficial to add foods that appear less healthy. This also may be for a shorter period until you can adjust your eating habits. Work with your registered dietitian to find the best nutrition plan for you.

Tips for Adding Calories

- ✓ Drizzle olive or avocado oil on your meals or incorporate it into smoothies

- ✓ Add extra butter, sour cream, heavy cream, mayonnaise, cream cheese, or ghee to your food

- √ Add avocado to foods or consume guacamole with chips as a snack

- √ Incorporate creamy dressing, sauces, and dips to salads, sandwiches, and meals

- √ Add high-calorie granola to yogurt, ice cream, or fruit

- √ Top desserts with sweetened condensed milk or whipped cream (ice cream, cake, muffins)

Tips for Adding Protein

- √ Consume a variety of protein sources (chicken, pork, beef, lamb, fish, eggs, dairy products, plant-based protein sources, and soy foods)

- √ Add protein or dry milk powders to smoothies, soups, oatmeal, or casseroles to boost the protein content

- √ Use nut butters to add protein to snacks (apples, bananas, toast, crackers)

- √ Snack on bean dips (hummus, white bean dip, black bean dip) with crackers, pita chips, pretzels, or vegetables

- √ Snack on seeds and whole nuts

- √ Add nuts to baked goods

- √ Consume eggs at multiple meals (quiche, frittata, omelet, French toast, pasta dishes)

- √ Top dishes with extra cheese

12

- ✓ Sip on bone broth or add it to soups and stews
- ✓ Add blended, soaked cashews, almonds, or walnuts to soups

High-Protein High-Calorie Snack Ideas

Including calorie-rich snacks during the day is a good way to give your body more calories, protein, vitamins, and minerals. Calorie-rich snacks throughout the day can also help combat early satiety, anorexia, or loss of appetite and help you reach your individual nutrition goals. Try to eat a small meal or snack every 2 to 3 hours.

Recommendations

- Siggis® or Chobani® yogurt drinks
- Nut butter (peanut, almond, cashew), banana, and honey on a waffle
- Hardboiled or scrambled eggs with veggies
- Greek yogurt with granola and fresh or canned fruit
- Graham crackers with cream cheese and jelly
- Cottage cheese with berries or apples/cinnamon
- Cheese sticks or BabyBel™ cheese with crackers
- Hummus or bean dip with crackers or cut vegetables
- Guacamole or salsa with crackers or cut veggies
- English muffin toasted with mozzarella and tomato sauce

- Quesadilla with refried beans and cheddar or feta cheese (option to add tofu, chicken, or beef for additional protein)
- Oatmeal with apples/cinnamon or berries with nuts
- Bagel or crackers with cream cheese
- Cereal with whole milk or non-dairy milk alternative
- Tuna, chicken, or egg salad with avocado in a whole wheat pita or on crackers
- Roasted or dried beans, chickpeas for snacking

- Peanut butter and jelly sandwich
- Muffins, pumpkin, or banana bread with cream cheese
- Fruit cocktail cups (peach, pear, mandarin orange)
- Gogo Squeeze™ Applesauce
- Trail Mix (dried fruit, nuts, dry cereal, pumpkin seeds, sunflower seeds, coconut, etc.)
- Oatmeal with apples/cinnamon or berries (overnight oats are another great make-ahead snack idea)
- Ice cream, frozen yogurt, or pudding

12

Nausea and Vomiting

Nausea and vomiting can result from the cancer itself, side effects of chemotherapy, radiation therapy, immunotherapy, pain, psychological factors, and constipation. If left untreated, vomiting can lead to dehydration, electrolyte imbalances, weight loss, and vitamin/mineral deficiency. If you are undergoing chemotherapy and your prescribed chemotherapy regimen has a high risk of nausea/vomiting, your physician will prescribe anti-nausea and other medications to help manage these symptoms.

Tips to Manage Nausea and Vomiting

- √ Consume 5-6 smaller, more frequent meals throughout the day to help from getting too full or bloated.

- √ Avoid consuming liquids with solid foods. Try and consume liquids 30-60 minutes before or after meals.

- √ Eat slowly and chew thoroughly.

- √ Eat dry, bland foods to help settle your stomach (toast, crackers, pretzels). Keep these on hand or at your bedside to help manage symptoms.

- √ Consume room temperature or cold foods to reduce smell sensitivity.

- √ Avoid high-fat or creamy foods, which may be heavy for the stomach and take longer to digest.

- Avoid foods with strong spices or spicy heat.

- Utilize ginger ale, ginger chews, ginger teas, or ginger extract.

- Try sucking on Queasy Pops® to aid with nausea.

- Wear clothes that are not too tight to stay more comfortable.

- If nausea is associated with vomiting, keep yourself well hydrated with fluids and beverages with electrolytes (Gatorade®, Pedialyte®).

- If your physician prescribes anti-nausea medications during treatment, take them as directed. Time your prescription with your meals to ensure they work best.

- If the anti-nausea medications your physician has prescribed are not alleviating your nausea, contact your healthcare team. There are many anti-nausea medications available, and while one might not be helpful, it is likely another drug will.

- Contact your healthcare team if you are experiencing 4-5 episodes of nausea/vomiting in 24 hours.

12

Constipation

Constipation is the reduction of bowel movements or bowel movements that are hard to pass. This can be due to side effects of medications (chemotherapy, pain medications), diet, or dehydration.

Tips to Manage Constipation

- √ Aim for 25-35 grams of fiber each day, as tolerated.

- √ Choose whole grain bread and cereal rather than white bread and low-fiber cereal.

- √ Utilize hot beverages, hot cereal, or high-fiber foods to stimulate bowel movements.

- √ Incorporate probiotic-rich foods to help facilitate bowel movements.

- √ Choose quinoa, brown rice, or wild rice instead of white rice.

- √ When eating fresh fruits or vegetables, consume the skin for an additional fiber boost.

- √ Add more beans/legumes or lentils to soups and casseroles to boost the fiber content.

- √ Choose a variety of fresh fruit and vegetables to increase fiber in your diet instead of fruit juices without pulp.

- √ Aim to drink at least 8-12 cups of fluid per day.

- ✓ Drink prune juice or consume dried prunes to help promote bowel movements.

- ✓ Participate in medically appropriate physical activity to promote motility.

- ✓ If constipation persists, your physician may recommend over-the-counter medications or supplements to help alleviate symptoms.

Diarrhea

Diarrhea is the increase of three or more stools per day compared to usual or an increase in the liquidity of bowel movements that could be related to diet, emotional stress of treatment, intestinal irritation, medications (antibiotics, chemotherapy), radiation therapy, infection, or malabsorption.

Tips to Manage Diarrhea

- ✓ Consume smaller, more frequent meals throughout the day to help from getting too full or bloated

- ✓ Limit high-fiber food products. Refer to "Low-Fiber Diet" section for further information (page 42).

- ✓ Consume grains lower in fiber (refined white bread, cereals, rice, pasta, farina) to bulk stool.

- ✓ Consume fruits lower in fiber (applesauce, melon, cantaloupe, bananas) or use products such as Banatrol® to manage diarrhea.

- ✓ Avoid beverages with artificial sweeteners or sugar alcohols (sorbitol, xylitol, mannitol) as they may worsen symptoms.

- ✓ If your symptoms of diarrhea are related to malabsorption, refer to the Malabsorption section to learn more (page 54).

- ✓ Your doctor may prescribe or recommend over-the-counter medications to help manage diarrhea once infectious causes are ruled out.

- ✓ If you are having diarrhea, make sure you take in additional fluids to minimize the risk of dehydration.

Oral Rehydration Solutions (ORS)

ORS can be made with items at home or purchased (Pedialyte®, Ensure® Rapid Hydration Powder) and can be helpful to replace fluid loss. See the "Recipes" section for ORS that you can make at home.

Contact your healthcare team if you are experiencing 4-6 episodes of diarrhea in 24 hours.

Dry Mouth (Xerostomia)

Dry mouth or **xerostomia** is a complication of chemotherapy or radiation therapy and can cause issues with eating due to decreased saliva production causing taste alterations, thick, or ropy saliva. A dry mouth can also increase your risk of dental cavities.

Tips to Manage Dry Mouth

√ Consume small, frequent meals.

√ Alternate bites of foods with sips of the liquid.

√ Drink 8 to 12 cups of fluid each day to keep your mouth moist and loosen dry or thick saliva. Carry a water bottle to sip on liquids throughout the day.

√ Chew on carrots or celery, which have higher water content.

√ Limit caffeinated drinks such as coffee, tea, and colas which may worsen symptoms.

√ Moisten foods with additional sauces, gravies, broths, dressings, butters, or margarine.

√ Try and consume soft, moist proteins and avoid dry, chewy meats with gristle.

√ Try increasing saliva production by incorporating tart foods and drinks into your diet, such as lemonade or cranberry.

12

- √ Suck on frozen melons, grapes, popsicles, or ice chips to moisten your mouth.

- √ Chew on sugar-free gum and sugar-free lemon sucking candies to stimulate saliva.

- √ Use Xylimelts®, Biotene® rinse to help manage dry mouth.

- √ Avoid alcohol or alcohol-based mouthwashes, which may make dryness worse.

- √ Swish and spit with seltzer or club soda to help loosen and remove dry or thick saliva.

- √ Humidifiers can help moisten the air.

- √ Saliva substitutes or artificial saliva may also be helpful. Saliva substitutes are available over the counter or by prescription. Speak to your doctor or registered dietitian about what products may be right for you.

Taste and Smell Changes

Changes to taste and smell may accompany cancer or cancer treatments. These symptoms may be referred to as **dysgeusia**. Foods normally enjoyed may be unappealing and taste or smell different from day to day. Taste changes can vary from one person to another going through cancer treatments. Taste and smell are related, and smelling certain foods or flavors of

different foods may take your desire to eat that food away. Taste and smell changes may lead to difficulty eating and may result in weight loss and poor nutrition.

Tips to Manage Taste Changes

Try new or different foods you may not normally like. Pay attention to the foods and flavors you like. Try to add foods with these flavors more often into your diet. Avoid unappealing foods.

Good mouth care or oral care during treatment can help.

A homemade rinse of baking soda and salt can be used before and after meals and throughout the day for general mouth cleansing and to improve the sense of taste. Mix ¾ teaspoon of salt and 1 teaspoon of baking soda in 4 cups of water. Rinse your mouth with 1 cup 3-4 times a day.

Strategies for Managing Specific Taste Changes

Loss of Taste

- √ Add spices or seasonings to enhance the flavor of your food.

- √ Acidic foods like oranges and lemons may stimulate taste buds. Try Jell-O or beverages with these flavors but avoid if they irritate your mouth.

- √ Suck on sugar-free tart candies before or after a meal.

- √ Blend fresh fruits into smoothies, shakes, or yogurts.

- √ Try frozen fruits such as grapes or chopped melon.

- √ Eat fresh vegetables, which may be more appealing than canned.

- √ Marinate meats in acidic juices such as marinades containing sweet and sour, lemon, or fruit flavors. Incorporate herbs and spices, pickles, or other seasonings to foods.

Salty, Bitter, or Metallic taste

- √ Use spices or seasonings like onion, garlic, or chili powder. If foods taste too salty, add sweeteners or a small amount of sugar.

- √ Use low-sodium products to minimize added salts to foods.

- √ Avoid salty or acidic foods.

- √ Utilize plastic or bamboo utensils in place of metal utensils.

- √ Try sugar-free lemon drops, gums, or star mints.

- √ Try Metaqil® mouth rinse 3 times daily as needed.

Meats Taste Bitter or Strange

- √ Try other protein-rich foods like eggs, dairy products, beans, tofu, or soy-based products.

- √ Add marinades, sauces, and dressing to meat to adjust flavors.

- √ Choose chicken, turkey, eggs, dairy products, or mild-tasting/smelling fish if red meat tastes or smells strong.

12

Foods or Drinks Smell Unpleasant

- √ Choose cold or room-temperature foods instead of hot foods such as cold sandwiches, cheese, and crackers, yogurts, shakes/smoothies.

- √ Avoid the kitchen when food is being prepared.

- √ Eat in a well-ventilated area, turn on a kitchen fan, and cover foods when cooking.

- √ Cook outdoors.

- √ Avoid using a microwave which can spread odors.

- √ Use a straw and use a lid to cover your drink to avoid smells.

Sore Mouth or Throat

Cancer treatments such as chemotherapy can cause mouth irritation such as mouth sores or an inflamed mouth or throat. This is referred to as **mucositis**. Fungal infections such as thrush may occur. These issues can lead to inadequate food intake, dehydration, and weight loss. Taking good care of your mouth prevents bacteria buildup that can cause infections in the mouth and throat. The following food suggestions and tips can lessen discomfort and improve nutrition.

Tips for Managing Sore Mouth or Throat

√ Practice good oral care. Use a baking soda/salt rinse (see recipe on page 75) before and after meals and throughout the day. Avoid using dentures, if possible, especially if they do not fit well.

√ Eat soft foods such as mashed potatoes, cottage cheese, macaroni and cheese, and scrambled eggs.

√ Drink cold foods to soothe the mouth.

√ Suck on ice chips or popsicles.

√ Eat frozen fruits or mix in smoothies. Choose low-acid frozen fruits such as peaches or bananas.

√ Drink through a straw.

√ Avoid carbonated beverages.

√ Moisten or dunk bread in broths, soups, or gravy.

√ Use a blender to puree foods.

√ Make sure to eat high-calorie, high-protein foods to speed up healing time. Protein shakes can be used to help meet calorie and protein needs.

√ Use mild, non-alcohol-based mouth rinses.

√ Avoid smoking, chewing tobacco, or drinking alcohol.

√ Ask your medical team about any prescription mouth rinses that may help with discomfort.

Foods to Avoid with Sore Mouth or Throat

Acidic foods such as	oranges, lemons, limes, grapefruit, pineapple, kiwi, and tomatoes
Irritating spices such as	pepper, nutmeg, chili powder, and cloves
Sauces that are vinegar-based and/or spicy such as	hot sauce or oil and vinegar dressings
Crunchy or hard foods such as	bread, chips, crackers, or pretzels
Foods or drinks that are hot in temperature	
Alcohol and carbonated beverages	

12

Oral Thrush (Candidiasis)

Oral **thrush** is a fungal infection that may happen due to treatment or a weakened immune system. It can cause pain with swallowing, taste changes, and sore mouth. Your tongue may be coated with a white layer.

Tips for Managing Oral Thrush

- √ Practice good oral hygiene. Use baking soda/salt rinses. (page 75).

- √ Choose soft, low-acid foods and follow the above guidelines on best food choices.

- √ Avoid sugar and yeast derived foods.

- √ Ask your dietitian about probiotics.

- √ Ask your medical team for medications to ease discomfort or treat the infection.

- √ Hold 1 tablespoon of yogurt in your mouth for 5 minutes daily.

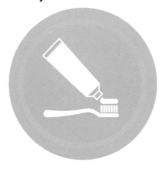

Gastroesophageal Reflux Disease (GERD)

Gastroesophageal Reflux Disease is a condition where the contents of the stomach flow back into the esophagus. It can cause heartburn or a burning sensation in your chest. It can worsen after meals or with lying down. Speak with your medical team if you are unable to control your symptoms with diet and lifestyle changes or over-the-counter medications.

Common GERD "Trigger" Foods

Carbonated beverages
Chocolate
Citrus fruits and juices containing orange, lemon, grapefruit, and pineapple
Coffee
Fatty, spicy, or greasy foods
Garlic
Peppermint or spearmint
Tomatoes/tomato products such as tomato sauces or tomato paste

12

Tips to Help Manage GERD

- √ Eat slowly in a relaxed environment. Allow at least 30 minutes for mealtime.

- √ Sit upright for an hour after eating.

- √ Take a 15-minute walk or move around after eating.

- √ Wear loose-fitting clothes.

- √ Wait for 3 hours after eating before laying down.

- √ Raise the head of your bed 6-9 inches.

- √ Avoid alcohol and tobacco products.

Gas and Bloating

There can be many causes of gas or bloating. Diet changes can help alleviate uncomfortable feelings of gas.

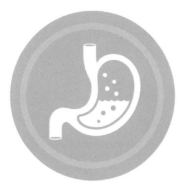

Tips for Managing Gas and Bloating

Limit or avoid consuming gas-producing foods:

Vegetables	broccoli, onions, garlic, cauliflower, cabbage, brussels sprouts, corn, radishes
Fruits	melons, apples, avocado
Others	beans/legumes, lentils, popcorn, fish, eggs, beef, dairy products, nuts

√ Avoid carbonated drinks, chewing gum, drinking through a straw.

√ Avoid sugar alcohols, which are typically found in "sugar-free" (sorbitol, maltitol, mannitol, xylitol) or no sugar added products such as gums, candies, and ice cream.

√ Eat small, frequent meals.

√ Consider over-the-counter products such as **Beano**® or **Simethicone** (Gas X® or Phazyme®).

√ Try ginger, peppermint, or fennel teas or candies to ease gas discomfort.

√ Exercise or move as able.

12

Lactose Intolerance

Lactose intolerance is a digestive disorder where the body does not make enough of the enzyme **lactase** to break down **lactose**, a naturally occurring sugar found in dairy products. If you have lactose intolerance, gas, bloating, abdominal discomfort, and diarrhea can occur after eating milk or dairy products. These symptoms may occur within 30 minutes to 2 hours after eating lactose-containing food or drinks.

> **Lactose intolerance can be present at birth or can develop over time.**

Inflammation, surgeries involving the digestive tract, chemotherapy treatments, and antibiotics can also cause lactose intolerance. Lactose tolerance can also differ between individuals, with some being able to tolerate more lactose than others.

Tips to Help with Lactose Intolerance

√ Try taking a lactase enzyme (such as Lactaid®) before eating milk or dairy products.

√ Look for "lactose-free" products in the dairy section of your grocery store.

√ Choose non-dairy milk alternatives such as soy, almond, oat, or non-dairy creamers instead of cow's milk.

√ Try small amounts of lactose-containing products to assess tolerance. Cultured dairy products such as yogurt and buttermilk may be easier to tolerate.

Cold Sensitivity

Oxaliplatin (Eloxitan®) is a chemotherapy medication that may be used in patients with cholangiocarcinoma. Oxaliplatin (Eloxitan®) can temporarily make individuals extra sensitive to cold. It is advised that patients follow tips to minimize cold exposure for at least 5 days following treatment to reduce the risk of side effects.

12

Side Effects of Cold Exposure

√ Tingling, numbness, stiffness, or tightness in hands and feet

√ Tightness in the throat or jaw (jaw spasms)

√ Difficulty swallowing

√ Abnormal tongue sensation

√ Difficulty breathing

√ Chest pressure

√ Nausea, vomiting, diarrhea

Tips for Managing Cold Sensitivity

- ✓ Wear gloves when taking items from the freezer or refrigerator.

- ✓ Drink through a straw.

- ✓ Do not use ice cubes or ice packs. Do not add ice to drinks.

- ✓ Do not eat or drink cold or frozen foods or drink cold beverages.

- ✓ Avoid ice cream and frozen treats such as popsicles or Italian ice.

- ✓ Cover your skin, nose, and mouth if it is cold outside.

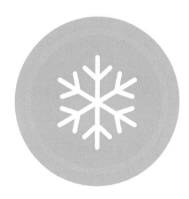

Warm Food Substitution List

The following list of foods can help guide food choices to help minimize cold sensitivities.

Instead of	Try
Cold beverages such as juice, soft drinks	Room temperature beverages such as fruit juices, lemonade, or teas
Refrigerated fruit	Room temperature fruit such as melon, grapes, apples, oranges
Cold high-calorie/protein supplements or shakes	Room temperature or warm "hot-chocolate style"
Popsicles	Lollipops, sugar-free hard candies, gelatin
Ice cream/sherbet	Warm custard, flan, pudding
Cereal with cold milk or non-dairy milk alternative	Warm oatmeal or Cream of Wheat® or Farina® made with milk or non-dairy milk alternative

12

Fatigue

Fatigue or a lack of energy is one of the most common side effects reported for cancer patients. It can be from the cancer itself or cancer treatments. Fatigue may result in poor eating, weight loss, or weight gain.

Tips for Managing Fatigue

- √ Stock your kitchen with easy-to-prepare and easy-to-eat foods (see list of foods below).

- √ Prepare meals on days when you feel your best and freeze meal-sized portions to have meals on hand on low-energy days.

- √ Keep snacks, **oral supplements,** and other prepared foods in the front of your refrigerator for easy access.

- √ Drink plenty of fluids as dehydration can make fatigue worse. Hydrating fluids include water, **oral rehydration solutions**, sports drinks, fruit juices, broth, or weak tea. Aim for 8-12 cups of fluids per day. If you are experiencing diarrhea, your fluid needs are higher (try to consume 1 additional cup of fluid per episode of diarrhea).

- √ Do not forget to eat. Try small, frequent meals.

- √ Consume foods that are softer and easy to chew.

- √ Limit consumption of caffeinated drinks such as coffee or tea to two cups per day.

√ Consume caffeinated drinks earlier in the day, so they don't interfere with sleep.

√ Keep non-perishable snacks at the bedside (such as small packages of nuts, trail mix, dried fruit)

√ Accept meals from friends and family members. Consider utilizing meal delivery services such as **Meals on Wheels** https://www. mealsonwheelsamerica.org/, **Mom's Meals** https:// www.momsmeals.com/, or another home/online delivery meal program.

√ Increase your physical activity level, as able, to help fight fatigue.

Easy to prepare and Eat Food List

The following foods are easy to prepare and can help you maintain your nutrition needs and reduce fatigue:

- Fresh seasonal fruits and vegetables
- Yogurt
- Pudding
- Applesauce
- Fruit cups
- Cheese sticks
- Nuts and seeds
- Trail mix
- Hummus
- Pretzels
- Hard-boiled eggs
- Popcorn
- Dried fruit
- Gelatin
- Protein or granola bars
- Crackers
- Frozen foods (microwaveable bags of vegetables, soups, casseroles)

- Potatoes (refrigerated, boxed mixes)
- Bakery items (muffins, pastries, pies, cookies, cakes)
- Oatmeal packets
- Whole grain cereals
- Pasta salad, chicken salad, tuna salad, egg salad
- Non-caffeinated beverages (fruit juice, sports drinks, protein shakes, bottled water, lemonade, pre-made smoothies, oral rehydration drinks)

Iron Deficiency

Iron carries oxygen throughout your body. Many factors may cause iron deficiency, including cancer itself or cancer treatments such as surgery or chemotherapy. Poor absorption or intake of iron and blood loss can also contribute to iron deficiency. You may feel tired and run down if you are deficient in iron. Dizziness, trouble maintaining body heat, pale skin, headache can all result from iron deficiency. Knowing how to maximize iron absorption through various food strategies and eating iron-rich foods can help improve iron deficiency.

Normal Iron Requirements
(Milligrams (mg)/day) for Healthy People

Age in years	Female	Male
19-50	18mg	8mg
51 & older	8mg	8mg

Tips for Increasing Iron in the Diet

√ Limit consumption of coffee, tea, and milk at mealtimes.

√ Look for cereals that are fortified with 100% of your daily value of iron, such as bran flakes.

√ Eat **enriched** or **fortified** grain products such as oatmeal, Cream of Wheat®, bread, and pasta.

√ Iron found in meats is called heme iron. **Heme iron** is better absorbed than iron in found plant foods, called **non-heme iron**. If possible, try to incorporate more sources of heme iron into your diet.

√ Eat foods that contain vitamin C. Vitamin C enhances the absorption of both heme and non-heme iron. Eat meat, poultry, and seafood with vitamin C-rich foods such citrus juice/fruits, peppers, strawberries, broccoli, and potatoes.

12

Good *Sources* of Iron

Lean meats and seafood provide the richest amounts of heme Iron. Nuts, beans, vegetables, and fortified grain products are good sources of non-heme iron.

Food	Servng Size	Iron Content
Breakfast cereals, fortified with 100% of daily value	1 serving	18mg
Oysters	3 ounces	8mg
White beans, canned	1 cup	8mg
Dark chocolate (45-69% cacao)	3 ounces	7mg
Beef liver	3 ounces	5mg
Lentils	1/2 cup	3mg
Spinach	1/2 cup	3mg
Tofu	1/2 cup	3mg
Oatmeal, fortified	1 cup, uncooked	3mg
Chickpeas, kidney beans	1/2 cup	2mg
Sardines with bone	3 ounces	2mg
Tomatoes, canned	1/2 cup	2mg
Beef, veal	3 ounces	2mg
Baked potato with skin	1 medium	2mg
Cashews	18 nuts	2mg
Dried prunes	4	2mg

High-Phosphorus (Hyperphosphatemia)

Genetic testing can provide access for patients with cholangiocarcinoma to effective, personalized treatment options. One in 5 cases of cholangiocarcinoma may have an FGFR2 mutation. These mutations may be treated with targeted therapies, which can cause high-phosphorus levels. High-phosphorus levels are found through lab work/blood tests.

> **Normal blood phosphorus levels are 2.8 to 4.5 mg/dL**

Phosphorus is an important mineral in the body. It helps build healthy bones and teeth and aids in nerve function and muscle movement. What you eat and drink can affect phosphorus levels in the body.

Tips for Reducing Phosphorus in the Diet

- √ Limit high-phosphorus foods. Phosphorus is naturally occurring in meats, dairy, and grains. Please refer to "Phosphorus Foods List" on the next page for a list of these foods.

- √ Buy fresh produce, unseasoned whole grains, nuts, lentils, seeds, and beans.

- √ Phosphorus can be added as a preservative to foods. Read ingredient lists on food to check for **phosphorus additives**. Ingredients that include "phos" indicate phosphorus has been added. Examples include

phosphoric acid, sodium **phos**phate, sodium hexameta**phos**phate, dicalcium **phos**phate.

√ Foods with the highest added phosphate include processed foods, beverages, and fast foods.

√ You may be advised to take a phosphorus binder to take with meals and snacks. A low-phosphorus diet is necessary for phosphorus binders to work correctly.

√ Discuss any over-the-counter products you take with your physician as they may interact with other medications.

Nutrition Facts

32 servings per container

Serving size	**3 g**

Amount Per Serving

Calories 150

	% Daily Value*
Total Fat 6g	8%
Saturated Fat 1g	5%
Trans Fat 0g	
Cholesterol 0mg	0%
Sodium 440mg	19%
Total Carbohydrate 24g	9%
Dietary Fiber 2g	7%
Total Sugars 0g	
Includes 0g Added Sugars	0%
Protein 2g	4%
Vitamin D 0mcg	0%
Calcium 1014mg	80%
Iron 0.0648mg	0%
Potassium 470mg	10%
Phosphorus	8%

* The % Daily Value (DV) tells you how much a nutrient in a serving of food contributes to a daily diet. 2,000 calories a day is used for general nutrition advice.

INGREDIENTS: POTATOES, VEGETABLE OIL (SUNFLOWER, COTTTONSEED, SOYBEAN AND/OR CANOLA), MODIFIED FOOD STARCH, RICE FLOUR, SALT, DEXTRIN, CORNSTARCH, LEVENING (SODIUM ACID PYROPHOSPHATE, SODIUM BARCARBONATE), DEXTROSE, XANTHAM GUM, ANNATO (COLOR), DISODIUM DIHYDROGEN PYROPHOSPHATE.

12

√ Stay well-hydrated – drink 8 to 12 cups of fluid every day.

√ Exercise as able.

Phosphorus Foods List

High-Phosphorus Foods	
Processed meats such as bacon, ham, hotdogs, chicken nuggets/strips, bologna, salami, sausage	Fresh or frozen potatoes or vegetables with "phos" ingredients
Organ meats such as kidney or liver	Frozen or canned fruits with "phos" ingredients or added sauces
Breaded, battered, or fried chicken, fish, or seafood	Meals or soups with less than 600 mg of sodium per serving and "phos" ingredients
Non-dairy creamers, enriched almond, or rice milk	Powdered mixes with "phos" ingredients
Processed cheese products or spreads such as American cheese slices, Velveeta™, CheezWhiz™, cream cheese	Coke™, Pepsi™ or Dr. Pepper™, energy/sports drinks, flavored waters, Crystal Light™ (grape, fruit punch, orange, raspberry flavors)
Ice cream, pudding, yogurt, frozen yogurt	Canned or bottled coffee or tea
Processed bread, oatmeal, cereals with "phos" ingredients on the label	Wine or beer

Low-Phosphorus Foods

All-natural chicken, fish, or seafood	Natural cheese such as brie, Swiss, cheddar, mozzarella, or feta (limit to 1 ounce)
Lean and fresh beef, pork, veal	Sherbet, sorbet, fruit ice, popsicles
Cottage cheese, sour cream, low-fat cream cheese, or dairy with no "phos" ingredients added	Fresh bread, bagels, English muffins, or pitas with no "phos" ingredients
Whole eggs or egg whites	Sprite™, 7-Up™, Sierra Mist™
Tofu, lentils, beans, hummus (limit to 1/3-1/4 cup)	Fresh, frozen, or canned vegetables without added "phos" ingredients
Unsalted nuts (1/4 cup) or nut butters (1 tbsp)	Meals or soups with more than 600 mg of sodium per serving and no "phos" ingredients
Milk, unenriched almond, or rice milk (limit ½ cup)	Water
Fresh lemonade, Crystal Light™ (lemonade, green tea, tea flavors), AriZona™ or Pure Leaf™ teas	Reduced salt crackers, rice cakes, pretzels, popcorn, or tortilla chips with no "phos" ingredients
Freshly brewed coffee or tea made from coffee beans, powdered coffee, or tea bags	

12

Food Safety

Depending on your individualized cancer treatment, there may be times that your immune system may not be able to help fight off harmful germs from your environment or even the foods you are eating. During these times, it is important to ensure that you are following food safety practices to keep yourself safe and decrease your risk of infection from foodborne illnesses.

Food Safety Tips

√ Always wash your hands for 20 seconds with hot, soapy water before preparing or eating food.

√ Foodborne illnesses are not visible to the naked eye and cannot be identified by smelling or tasting foods. You should never taste food to determine if it is safe.

√ Keep hot foods hot and cold foods cold.

√ Avoid communal food from buffets and salad bars. Never buy food displayed in unsafe or unclean conditions.

√ Take care to wash fresh fruits and vegetables in warm water before peeling, cutting, or consuming. You do not need to use liquid soap, detergents, or vegetable wash; plain water should suffice. Dry after washing with a clean cloth.

√ Avoid eating pre-cut fruits and vegetables.

√ Heat deli meats and hot dogs before eating.

√ Avoid raw seafood such as sushi, sashimi, raw oysters, clams, scallops, or ceviche. Raw seafood may contain parasites and bacteria that could make you ill.

√ Choose pasteurized juice, cider, and dairy products. Dairy products that have been pasteurized will state "Grade A" on the label.

√ If you are unsure of the safety of a food item, do not take the risk. The golden rule of food safety is *"when in doubt, throw it out."*

13

√ Reach out to your treatment team and registered dietitian if you have specific questions about your food choices.

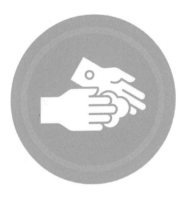

4 Basic Steps of Food Safety

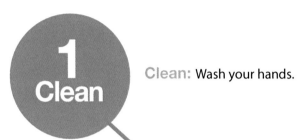

Clean: Wash your hands.

Separate: Keep raw and cooked foods and their juices away from each other.

3 Cook

Cook: Cook proteins and eggs to safe temperatures to eliminate illness-causing pathogens they may contain:

- Turkey, fish, poultry: 165°F
- Ground meats (beef, veal, pork, lamb): 145°F
- Eggs/egg dishes: 160°F
- Steak, roasts, chops (beef, veal, pork, lamb): 145° F
- Fish and seafood: 145°F

4 Chill

Chill: Chill foods within 2 hours of preparation or purchasing, 1 hour if temperatures are above 90°F. Avoid eating foods that have been sitting out as this allows bacteria to collect. Keep your refrigerator at 40 °F.

Oral Supplements

If you are eating less than expected, oral supplements may be beneficial to help you achieve your individualized calorie and protein requirements during treatment. Below is a list of shakes that you can try and incorporate into your diet. They have extra calories, protein, and nutrients to maintain weight, strength, and energy. Most shakes can be found at grocery stores, pharmacies, or online. Shakes can be consumed at room temperature, chilled, or combined with other foods to increase further the calories and protein they provide. Talk to your doctor or registered dietitian about what oral supplement or nutritional shake is right for you.

Commercially Available Oral Supplement Shakes List

High-Calorie High-Protein Shakes (Whey Protein Based)

- Ensure Enlive® (8 ounces): 350 calories, 20 g protein
- Ensure Max Protein® (8 ounces): 150 calories, 30 g protein, 1 gram sugar
- Boost® Original (8 ounces): 240 calories, 10 g protein
- Boost® Max Protein (11 ounces): 160 calories, 30 g protein, 1 gram sugar
- Boost® Very High Calorie (8 ounces): 530 calories, 22 g protein
- Enu™ (8.5 ounces): 340 calories, 17 g protein

Plant-Based, Protein-Based Shakes

- Orgain™ (11 ounces): 255 calories, 16 g protein
- Kate Farms® 1.4 Shake (11 ounces): 455 calories, 20 g protein
- Kate Farms® Nutrition Shake (11 ounces): 330 calories, 16 g protein
- Soylent® (14 ounces): 400 calories, 20 g protein, 1 g sugar
- OWYN Meal Replacer Shake™ (12 ounces): 300 calories, 20 g protein, 0 g sugar
- Ensure Plant-Based Protein® (11 ounces): 180 calories, 20 g protein

High-Calorie, High-Protein Powders (Flavored)

14

- ScandiShake® (8 ounces, mixed with whole milk): 600 calories, 12 g protein
- Carnation Instant Breakfast® (8 ounces): 280 calories, 12 g protein

Specialty Shakes

- Glucerna® for Glycemic Control (8 ounces): 180 calories, 10 g protein, 4 grams sugar
- Boost Glucose Control® (8 ounces): 190 calories, 16 g protein, 4 g sugar
- Premier Protein® (11 ounces): 160 calories, 30 g protein, 1 gram sugar

- Nepro® for Poor Kidney Function (8 ounces): 420 calories, 19 g protein, 225 mg potassium, 170 mg phosphorus
- MightyShakes® Nectar Consistency (8.5 ounces): 500 calories, 23 g protein

Juice Drinks (Fat-free, Potassium and Phosphorus Free)

- Ensure Clear® (8 ounces): 250 calories, 9 g protein
- Boost Breeze® (8 ounces): 250 calories, 9 g protein
- Boost Soothe® (8 ounces): 300 calories, 10 g protein
- VidaFuel® (2 ounces): 90 calories, 16 g protein

Ideas for Smoothie or Supplement Add-ins:

- Benecalorie® Unflavored (1.5 ounces): 330 calories, 7 g protein
- Powdered Peanut Butter PB2® (2 tablespoons): 45 calories, 5 g protein
- Vanilla ice cream (½ cup): 140 calories, 2 grams protein
- Unsweetened canned coconut milk (⅓ cup): 120 calories, <1 g protein

Of note, reference of any specific product does not constitute an endorsement, recommendation, or favoring by the Cholangiocarcinoma Foundation.

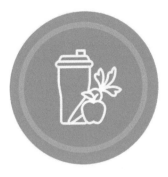

14

Complementary and Alternative Medicine (CAM

Complementary treatments are used in combination with standard cancer treatments and can include:

- Yoga
- Massage
- Acupuncture
- Reiki
- Meditation
- Aromatherapy and others

Alternative treatments are used in place of standard cancer treatments and may not have research to confirm their effectiveness.

Because research is often limited for CAM therapies, it is important to talk to your doctor about any complementary treatments you are considering, as they can interact with or change the effectiveness of your primary treatment. Some complementary therapies, such as yoga and acupuncture, have been studied for use in cancer patients to help reduce side effects when used alongside standard medical treatments.

Try aromatherapy for nausea by placing a few drops of peppermint essential oil on a cotton ball and leave on a table or surface near where you are sitting.

For more information on CAM, you can visit:

https://cam.cancer.gov/

https://www.nccih.nih.gov/

15

Vitamin and Mineral Supplements

Dietary supplements are typically in pill, capsule, or powder form and are intended to add specific nutrients to the diet. They may include vitamins, minerals, herbs, botanicals, or other components. Vitamins and other supplements may interact with treatments for cholangiocarcinoma. It is recommended to avoid high doses of antioxidant supplements (such as vitamin A, C, and E) during chemotherapy and radiation treatments. It is best to talk with your doctor and dietitian about any supplements that interact with your specific treatment. Always aim to meet your vitamin, mineral, and antioxidant needs through food, as able.

> **Check with your doctor or dietitian before starting any new supplements, as many may interact with your prescribed treatment regimen or have side effects.**

Supplements may be needed in certain cases for patients with cholangiocarcinoma, especially if you have had surgery on your digestive tract or if you have limited certain food groups in your diet. For example, patients with fat malabsorption may be at greater risk for deficiencies in vitamins A, D, E, and K. Patients with **anemia** may require supplementation of iron, folic acid, or vitamin B12. The safest way to supplement these nutrients in your diet is by talking with your oncologist and registered dietitian about regularly monitoring these nutrients' levels with lab tests.

Vitamin and Mineral Supplement Safety

Over-the-counter (OTC) supplements are not well regulated in the United States. Claims made on supplement labels may not be supported by research and are required to include a disclaimer that it has not been evaluated by the Food and Drug Administration (FDA).

> * These statements have not been evaluated by the Food and Drug Administration. This product is not intended to diagnose, treat, cure or prevent any disease.

In random testing, some supplements have been found to have higher or lower levels of nutrients than what is advertised or may contain high levels of contaminants. Some supplement companies pay for independent party verification to avoid this, such as the United States Pharmacopeial Convention (USP®) or National Sanitation Foundation (NSF®) verification.

16

Taking OTC supplements in large doses may also cause digestive upset like nausea or diarrhea. In some cases, the body processes these supplements in a similar way to your medications or cancer treatment, which can increase or decrease that medication's effectiveness. In many cases, a well-balanced diet can meet vitamin and mineral needs. It is best to speak with your registered dietitian regarding whether supplements are necessary and safe to take during or after treatment.

For more information on supplement safety, you can visit:

https://ods.od.nih.gov/

https://www.fda.gov/food/dietary-supplements

Conclusion

This resource was written and developed for cholangiocarcinoma patients by certified cancer dieticians. For more information and resources, please visit the Foundation website at:

https://cholangiocarcinoma.org/

Cholangiocarcinoma Foundation
5526 West 13400 South, #510
Herriman, Utah 84096 U.S.A.

(888) 936-6731
info@cholangiocarcinoma.org

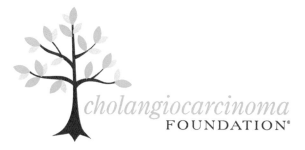

Patients
First

Recipes

Each healthy, nourishing recipe below corresponds with the meal plans above (low-fat and low-fiber diets).
Asterisks (*) indicate tips and additions for recipes. It is important to stay mindful of ingredients and suggestions when reading notes. Some additional notes may not comply with diet instructions; however, each original recipe is safe to consume with the matching meal menu.

Many of these meals can be made ahead of time and then eaten as leftovers throughout the week. Refrigerate or freeze in individual containers to reduce fatigue from cooking. Of note, monitor time left in the fridge and make sure to adhere to food safety practices.

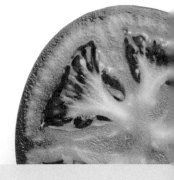

116

Open-Faced Tuna Melt

Yields 4 servings
Total time: 30 minutes

- 4 slices whole grain bread
- 1 can (5 ounces) tuna in water, drained
- 2 teaspoons lemon juice
- 2 tablespoons hummus
- 1 tomato, thinly sliced
- 8 ounces low-fat mozzarella cheese, shredded
- Salt and pepper, to taste

1   In a bowl, add tuna and break apart. Add lemon juice, hummus, salt, and pepper; mix until combined.

2   Under the broiler or in a toaster oven, toast the bread until golden brown. Remove from the oven.

3   Top each slice of bread with about a ½ cup tuna salad, 2 tomato slices, and 2 ounces of shredded cheese.

4   Place back under the broiler or in the toaster oven until cheese melts, about 3-5 minutes.

*   Substitute mozzarella or other cheese of choice
*   Add pickles, capers, or olives to tuna salad for extra flavor

Sheet Pan Chicken Fajitas

Yields 6 servings
Total Time: 35 minutes

- 1 pound chicken breast, boneless, skinless, thinly sliced
- 1 large bell pepper, any color, sliced
- 1 large onion, sliced
- 1 ½ teaspoons cumin
- ½ teaspoon dried oregano
- 1 teaspoon chili powder
- 1 teaspoon garlic powder
- 1 teaspoon salt
- ¼ teaspoon ground black pepper
- 1 tablespoon olive oil
- 1 lime, halved
- 6 flour tortillas

1   Preheat the oven to 400 degrees Fahrenheit. Cover a baking sheet (18 by 13 inches) with aluminum foil.

2   Place sliced chicken breast, sliced bell pepper, and sliced onion in a bowl. Sprinkle it with cumin, dried oregano, chili powder, garlic powder, salt, and black pepper. Add olive oil. Toss until seasonings are evenly distributed.

3   Spread the chicken, peppers, and onion mixture onto a baking sheet. Make sure to spread in an even layer to help it cook consistently.

4   Roast in the oven for 18-25 minutes and mix halfway through cooking. Bake until the vegetables are tender

and the chicken has reached an internal temperature of 165 degrees Fahrenheit.

5   When fajita filling is taken out of the oven, squeeze fresh lime juice over the top.

6   Place fajita filling in flour tortillas and add toppings of choice.

   ✳   Top with low-fat shredded cheese, salsa, or non-fat Greek yogurt

Corn Salad

Yields 4 servings
Total Time: 20 minutes

- 4 cups corn (defrosted from frozen or fresh)
- ½ cup red onion, diced
- ½ cup cherry tomatoes, quartered
- 1 tablespoon lime juice
- 1 tablespoon olive oil
- 1 garlic clove, minced
- ½ teaspoon salt
- ½ teaspoon ground black pepper
- ½ cup fresh cilantro, chopped

1   Whisk together lime juice, olive oil, garlic, salt, and pepper in a bowl.

2   Add corn, onion, tomato, and cilantro. Mix until combined.

   ✳   To spice up the salad, add ½ a minced jalapeño.
   ✳   For a different flavor profile, exchange lime juice for apple cider vinegar and cilantro for basil.

Carrot Ginger Soup

Yields 4-6 servings
Total Time: 45-60 minutes

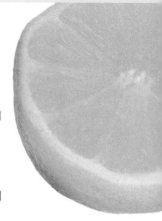

- 3 cups carrots, roughly chopped
- 1 large onion, diced
- 2 cloves garlic, chopped
- 1 tablespoon olive oil
- 2 teaspoons fresh ginger, grated
- 1 teaspoon turmeric, ground
- 1 tablespoon apple cider vinegar
- 4 cups vegetable broth
- 1 teaspoon salt
- ½ teaspoon ground black pepper

In a large pot, heat olive oil. Add onions, ginger, garlic and cook for 2 minutes or until the onion is translucent. Season with salt and pepper.

1 Add carrots and vegetable broth to the pot. Simmer the carrots until they are fork-tender, about 30 minutes.

2 Transfer the soup to the blender and blend until smooth. Make sure the soup is not too hot when it is added to the blender.

3 Place the blended soup back in the pot and adjust for seasoning.

* The amount of broth you add will determine soup thickness and consistency. More broth will make a thinner soup.
* Add a drizzle of coconut milk or heavy cream to make the soup creamy.
* Top with a dollop of pesto, toasted nuts, pumpkin seeds, herbs, or olive oil

Orzo with Lemon, Parmesan, and Shredded Chicken

Yields 4-6 servings
Total Time: 30 minutes

- 1 cup orzo
- 1 cup chicken broth
- ½ cup milk
- 1 tablespoon olive oil
- ¼ cup onion, chopped
- 1 garlic clove, minced
- ½ cup chicken breast, cooked, shredded
- 1 tablespoon lemon juice
- 1 teaspoon chopped parsley
- 1 ounce shredded parmesan
- Salt and pepper

1   Heat olive oil in a pan.

2   Sauté onion and garlic for 2 minutes until onion is translucent.

3   Add orzo and cook for 2 more minutes, frequently stirring until toasted.

4   Add the broth and milk; bring to a boil and then reduce to a simmer. Cook for 5 minutes.

5   Stir in shredded chicken, parmesan, parsley, and lemon juice. Season with additional salt and pepper as needed.

*   Milk can be substituted with cream, half and half, or unsweetened coconut milk for more calories.
*   Peas, spinach, broccoli, zucchini, squash, mushrooms, or asparagus can be added to increase vegetable content.
*   To add extra flavor and spice, add ½ a teaspoon of red pepper flakes.

Overnight Oatmeal

Yields 1 serving
Total Time: Two hours to overnight

- 1 cup old-fashioned rolled oats
- 1 cup almond milk
- 2 tablespoons blueberries
- 5 walnuts, chopped

1 Mix oats and almond milk in a glass jar or plastic container.

2 Top with blueberries and walnuts.

3 Leave in the refrigerator overnight (or for over 2 hours). Stir and enjoy.

* Use any milk, non-dairy milk alternative, or part yogurt
* Add any seeds, nuts, nut butter, fresh or dried fruit to customize the flavor
* Add any sweetener (honey, maple syrup, brown sugar, agave)

Egg Salad

Yields 1 serving
Total Time: 15 minutes

- 2 hard-boiled eggs, peeled and chopped
- 2 tablespoons mayonnaise
- 1 teaspoon Dijon mustard
- 1 teaspoon parsley, chopped
- Salt and pepper to taste

1 Place all ingredients in a bowl.

2 Mix well and serve with crackers or toast.

Smoothies

Add all ingredients to a blender and blend until smooth.

Peanut Butter Banana
337 calories, 13 g protein

- 1 banana, peeled
- 1 scoop protein powder
- 2 tablespoons peanut butter
- 1 tablespoon honey
- 1 cup milk
- 1 cup ice

Banana Blueberry
347 calories, 25 g protein

- 1 banana, peeled
- ½ cup blueberries, frozen
- 1 scoop protein powder
- 2 tablespoons almond butter
- ½ cup almond milk

Orange Crème
520 calories, 30 g protein

- 1 cup orange juice
- 1 scoop vanilla protein powder
- 3 tablespoons cashew butter
- ½ cup almond milk

Oral Rehydration Solutions to help replace fluid loss

Using Gatorade G2

- 1-liter G2 (4 ½ cups)
- ½ teaspoon salt

With Grape or Cranberry Juice

- ½ cup juice
- 3 ½ cups water
- ½ teaspoon salt

With Orange Juice

- ½ teaspoon salt
- ½ teaspoon baking soda
- 8 teaspoons sugar
- 1 cup unsweetened orange juice without pulp
- 1 liter of water (4½ cups)

With Chicken Broth

- 4 cups water
- 1 dry chicken broth cube
- ¼ teaspoon table salt
- 2 tablespoons sugar
  OR
- 2 cups chicken broth (not low sodium)
- 2 cups water
- 2 tablespoons sugar

World Health Organization Recipe

- 3/8 teaspoon salt (sodium chloride)
- ¼ teaspoon salt substitute (potassium chloride)
- ½ teaspoon baking soda (sodium bicarbonate)
- 2 tablespoons + 2 teaspoons sugar (sucrose)
- Add water to make one 1-liter (8 cups)
- Optional: Nutrasweet® or Splenda® based flavoring of choice, to taste

Oley Foundation Recipe

- ¾ teaspoon salt
- 1 tablespoon + 1 teaspoon sugar
- 2 cups Sprite Zero
- 1 envelope of orange or lemon sugar-free drink flavoring mix (for 2 cups)

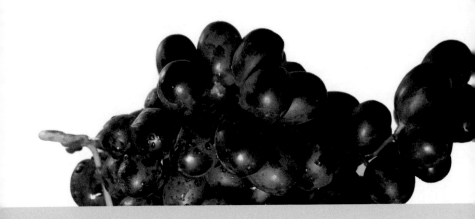

Resources

American Cancer Society
Reducing cancer risk, treatment, and recovery research.

https://www.cancer.org/

American Institute for Cancer Research
Cancer nutrition information, recipes, cookbooks, weekly recipes via email.

https://www.aicr.org/

Chemotherapy
View common symptoms and how to manage side effects of chemotherapy.

http://chemocare.com/
https://www.oncolink.org/

Radiation
Education about radiation therapy treatment.

https://www.astro.org/Patient-Care-and-Research/Patient-Education/Patient-Brochures
https://www.cancer.gov/publications/patient-education/radiationttherapy.pdf

Cholangiocarcinoma Foundation

Learn about our Programs and Services

Cholangiocarcinoma Overview
https://cholangiocarcinoma.org

Find a Local Specialist
https://cholangiocarcinoma.org/specialist-map/

Research the Latest Clinical Trials
https://cholangiocarcinoma.org/professionals/
research/clinical-trials/

Receive a Free e-Book
https://cholangiocarcinoma.org/publications/

Join our Monthly Patient and Caregiver Support Groups
https://cholangiocarcinoma.org/calendar/

Resources

Become a Mentor/Request a Mentor
https://cholangiocarcinoma.org/cholangioconnect/

Join the Patient Registry
https://cholangiocarcinoma.org/professionals/
research/patient-registry/

Learn why Biomarkers Matter

https://cholangiocarcinoma.org/mutationsmatter/
biomarkers-matter/

Academy of Nutrition and Dietetics
Science-based food and nutrition information.

https://www.eatright.org/

American Psychological Oncology Society
Assists patients and caregivers with resources, programs, and support to ease the cancer journey.

https://apos-society.org/

Cancer Care
Free professional support services (online, telephone, and in-person) for caregivers and loved ones as well as caregiving information and additional resources.

https://www.cancercare.org/

Cancer Hope Network

Volunteers provide free and confidential one-on-one telephone support for people with cancer and family members.

https://www.cancerhopenetwork.org/

Caregiver Action Network

Supports and educates family caregivers, helps them connect with other caregivers, and helps them become their own advocates. Membership is free to caregivers.

https://caregiveraction.org/

Complementary and Alternative Medicine

Education about complementary and alternative medicine.

https://cam.cancer.gov/
https://www.nccih.nih.gov/

Family Caregiver Alliance

Information and resources for long-term caregiving, including practical skills, how to hold family meetings, decision-making, assistive equipment, online support.

https://www.caregiver.org/

Resources

Meals on Wheels

A program which supports virtually every community in America and delivers nutritious meals to the nation's seniors.

https://www.mealsonwheelsamerica.org/

Mom's Meals

Mom's Meals offers menu options specifically tailored to meet the nutritional needs of cancer patients.

https://www.momsmeals.com/our-food/nutrition/cancer-support/

National Cancer Institute

Cancer basics and treatments.

https://www.cancer.gov/

NeedyMeds

A non-profit organization focused on making information about medical assistance programs available to those in need at no cost.

https://www.needymeds.org/

Oley Foundation

A resource for individuals receiving tube feeding or intravenous nutrition. Resources, support groups, and additional information can be found on their webpage.

https://oley.org/

Oncology Nutrition Dietetics Practice Group

Eating well when unwell. Healthy nutrition recipes, menus, and diets. Locate an Oncology Nutrition Specialist in your area.

https://www.oncologynutrition.org/home

Social Security Extra Help Plan

A program to help people with limited income and resources pay Medicare prescription drug program costs, like premiums, deductibles, and coinsurances.

https://www.ssa.gov/benefits/medicare/prescriptionhelp/

Vitamin/Mineral Supplement Safety

Reputable information on vitamins, minerals, and other dietary supplements.

https://www.fda.gov/food/dietary-supplements
https://ods.od.nih.gov/

Resources

Cookbooks

The Cancer-Fighting Kitchen Second Edition
Rebecca Katz (2010)

One Bite at a Time: Nourishing Recipes for Cancer Survivors and Their Friends
Mat Edelson and Rebecca Katz (2008)

American Cancer Society What to Eat During Cancer Treatment
Jeanne Besser, Kristina Ratley, RD, LDN, Sheri Knecht, MS, RD, LDN, Michele Szafranski, MS, RD, LDN (2009)

Betty Crocker Living with Cancer Cookbook
Kris Ghosh, MD, MBA and Linda Carson, MD (2011)

Eating Well Through Cancer
Holly Clegg and Gerald Miletello, MD (2006)

The New American Plate Cookbook: Recipes for a Healthy Weight and a Healthy Life
The American Institute for Cancer Research (2005)

The Essential Cancer Treatment Nutrition Guide & Cookbook
Jean LaMantia and Neil Berinstein (2012)

Cook for Your Life: Delicious, Nourishing Recipes for Before, During, and After Cancer Treatment
Ann Odgen Gaffney (2015)

American Cancer Society Complete Guide to Nutrition for Cancer Survivors
Barbara L Grant (2010)

Healing Gourmet Eat to Fight Cancer
Simin Liu, MD, Kathy McManus, RD, John A Carlio, CEC (2005)

The Cancer Lifeline Cookbook: Good Nutrition, Recipes, and Resources to Optimize the Lives of People Living with Cancer
Kimberly Mathai, MS, RD with Ginny Smith (2004)

The Cancer Survival Cookbook: 200 Quick and Easy Recipes with Helpful Eating Hints
Christina Marino, MD, MPH, Donna Weihoffen, RD, MS (1997)

The Cancer Wellness Cookbook: Smart Nutrition and Delicious Recipes for People Living with Cancer
Julia Hopper and Kimberly Mathia, MS, RD (2014)

Food For Thought-Healing Foods to Savor, Second Edition
Sheila Kealey, Vicky Newman, and Susan Faerber (2012)

Cooking with Foods that Fight Cancer
Richard Bèliveau, Ph. D and Denis Gingras, Ph. D. (2006)

Cookbooks

Glossary

Absorption: The movement of nutrients, water, and electrolytes from the gastrointestinal tract into the bloodstream.

Alternative Treatment: Treatments that are not regulated by the Food and Drug Administration because they are unproven and often promoted as cures used in place of standard treatment. Alternative therapies include the use of dietary supplements, special teas, vitamins, herbal preparations, and practices such as massage therapy, acupuncture, spiritual healing, and meditation.

Amylase: An enzyme secreted in saliva and by the pancreas that breaks down complex carbohydrates called starches.

Anemia: A condition in which the number of red blood cells is lower than normal.

Anorexia: The loss of appetite or desire to eat.

Beano®: A natural food enzyme that works with your body to break down complex carbohydrates in food (fresh fruits, vegetables, whole grains, beans, or legumes) to prevent gas before it starts and improve digestion.

Bicarbonate: Produced by the pancreas during digestion. Neutralizes acidic stomach contents entering the duodenum to allow for pancreatic enzymes to digest food.

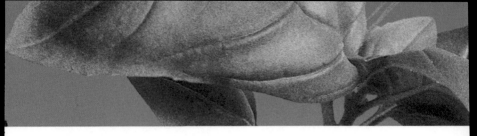

Bile: A fluid made by the liver and stored in the gallbladder. Bile is excreted into the small intestine where it helps digest fat in the diet.

Cachexia: A condition marked by weight loss and muscle loss due to the body's improper use of calories and proteins. Cancer-related cachexia creates fatigue and weakness and may impair the body's response to treatment.

Calories: Energy available in food.

Carbohydrate: A nutrient found in food. Carbohydrates are the preferred fuel for most body functions. With the exception of milk, foods high in carbohydrates are derived from plant sources.

Central Line: A type of IV that is inserted into a larger vein near the heart or just inside the heart to allow for patients to receive medications, fluids, blood products, or nutrition.

Complementary treatment: A type of treatment in which alternative therapies such as acupuncture, massage, reiki, or yoga are used in conjunction with conventional medicine to enhance care.

Chemotherapy: Drugs used to kill cancer cells in individuals with cancer. Can be used alone or in combination to treat a wide variety of cancers. Can be provided orally, topically, through an IV, or injection.

Glossary

Cholecystectomy: A surgery performed to remove the gallbladder.

Constipation: A condition characterized by hard, dry bowel movements. It is associated with discomfort in passing stools and/or infrequent passing of stools.

Corticosteroids: A type of medication that works to reduce inflammation in the body or immune system activity. Some may be used to help manage chemotherapy-induced nausea and vomiting.

Includes medications such as PredniSONE, Dexamethasone, MethylPREDNISone, Hydrocortisone.

Cyclosporin (Neoral®): Immunosuppressive medication used after transplant to prevent organ rejection.

Dehydration: Not having enough water, fluid, and electrolytes to maintain health, either due to decreased intake or excess losses.

Diabetes: A chronic disease that affects the body's ability to produce or properly use the hormone insulin. In type 1 diabetes, the pancreas does not produce insulin. In type 2 diabetes, the pancreas does not produce enough insulin, or the body does not use it properly.

Diarrhea: A condition marked by frequent and loose bowel movements.

Digestion: The process of breaking down food so that the body can use it.

Distal Cholangiocarcinoma: This type of cancer is found in the distal region. The distal region is made up of the common bile duct which passes through the pancreas and ends in the small intestine. Distal bile duct cancer is also called extrahepatic cholangiocarcinoma.

Distal Pancreatectomy: A type of pancreatic surgery where the body and tail of the pancreas and often the spleen is removed.

Duodenum: The first part of the intestine where food from the stomach mixes with bile from the gallbladder and digestive juices from the pancreas.

Duodenal Stent: A hollow tube placed into the duodenum to relieve obstruction or blockage and allow food and liquids to pass normally.

Dumping Syndrome: A condition in which there is rapid emptying of the stomach shortly after eating. It may be characterized by flushed skin, weakness, dizziness, abdominal pain, nausea, vomiting, and/or diarrhea.

Dysgeusia: Altered or impaired sense of taste.

Early Satiety: Feeling of being full after eating or drinking a small amount.

Glossary

Electrolytes: Electrically charged minerals that help to maintain (1) the proper amount and kind of fluid in every compartment of the body and (2) the acid-base (pH) balance of the body. Electrolytes include sodium, potassium, chloride, and magnesium.

Enriched Foods: Process in which nutrients lost during processing are added back to foods to restore the food to previous nutrient levels.

Enteral Nutrition: Nutrition, medications, or fluid provided into the gastrointestinal tract via a feeding tube, bypassing the mouth and sometimes the stomach.

Exocrine Pancreatic Insufficiency: A condition where the pancreas does not produce enough pancreatic enzymes to digest foods properly.

Extrahepatic Cholangiocarcinoma: This type of cancer forms in the bile ducts outside the liver. The extrahepatic bile duct is made up of the hilum region and the distal region.

Fat: The primary fuel source or storage form of energy in the body.

Fatigue: Lack of energy, tiredness, dizziness, or mental fuzziness caused by anemia, inadequate energy intake, protein intake, weight loss, pain, medications, anti-cancer treatment, dehydration, and/or sleep disturbances.

Fiber: Indigestible component of carbohydrates with health benefits, found in plant-based foods.

FGFR2 Mutation (fibroblast growth factor receptor 2): A genetic mutation that can occur in individuals with cholangiocarcinoma.

Fortified Foods: Foods that have nutrients added to them that typically do not occur in the food.

Furosemide (Lasix®): Diuretic medication used to increase water and salt excretion from the kidneys through urine.

Gastroesophageal Reflux Disease (GERD): Chronic disease that occurs when stomach contents flow back (reflux) into the food pipe (esophagus).

Gastrostomy Tube (G-Tube): A feeding tube inserted through the abdomen into the stomach. Special liquid food is given to the patient through the G-tube. Pancreatic enzymes may be incorporated to aid in the breakdown and absorption of nutrients.

Glucose: A simple sugar that provides a significant energy source for the body. Carbohydrates are broken down to form glucose for use by the body.

Heme Iron: Iron present in animal proteins such as meats, poultry, seafood, and fish that is well absorbed.

Glossary

Hemoglobin A1C: A blood test that measures your average blood sugar levels over 2-3 months. Used in the diagnosis of diabetes.

Hilar Cholangiocarcinoma: A type of bile duct cancer that occurs in the bile ducts that lead out of the liver (hepatic ducts) and join with the gallbladder.

Hydration: Getting the right amount of water, fluid, and electrolytes to maintain health.

Hyperkalemia: High potassium levels in the blood. Normal blood potassium levels are 3.5-5.1 mmol/L.

Hyperphosphatemia: Elevated levels of phosphorus in the blood. Normal blood phosphorus levels are 2.8 to 4.5 mg/dL.

Ileus: Lack of intestinal movement. It can occur after surgery or due to medications.

Immunotherapy: A type of cancer treatment that helps a person's immune system better recognize and destroy cancer cells.

Immunosuppressive: Decreases the ability of the body's immune system to fight infection or other diseases.

Insoluble Fiber: A tough, indigestible fiber that does not dissolve readily in water. Food sources include fruits, vegetables, seeds, nuts, legumes, and whole grains. Possible health effects of consuming insoluble fiber include softened stools, regulation of bowel movements, and lowered blood cholesterol.

Intrahepatic Cholangiocarcinoma: Intrahepatic CCA occurs inside the liver where cancer develops in the hepatic bile ducts or the smaller intrahepatic biliary ducts.

Jejunostomy tube (J-tube): A feeding tube inserted through the abdomen into the small intestine, bypassing the stomach. Special liquid food is given to the patient through the J-tube. Pancreatic enzymes may be incorporated to aid in the breakdown and absorption of nutrients.

Klatskin Tumor: An extra-hepatic cholangiocarcinoma arising in the junction of the main right or left hepatic ducts to form the common hepatic duct.

Lactase: The enzyme necessary to break down the sugar lactose.

Lactose: The natural sugar found in milk and milk products.

Lactose Intolerance: A condition in which the body's digestive system cannot completely break down lactose. It is often caused by insufficient amounts of lactase.

Lipase: An enzyme secreted by the pancreas that breaks down fats.

Localized: When cancer is contained in a specific part of the body.

Locally Advanced: When cancer has grown outside of the body part it started in but has not yet spread to other parts of the body.

Glossary

Malabsorption: Decreased ability of the body to digest and absorb nutrients, possibly caused by chemotherapy, surgery, medications, medical conditions, or infections that result in gas, bloating, gastrointestinal pain, and/or diarrhea.

Metastatic: When cancer cells break apart where the original cancer was located and travel through the blood/lymphatic system to other parts of the body.

Motility: The movement of the gastrointestinal tract to allow food to pass from the mouth through the stomach, intestines, colon, and out of the body.

Mucositis: Inflammation of the mouth results in a painful, irritated throat or a lump in the throat. It can cause indigestion, esophageal reflux, belching, feeling of fullness, and early satiety.

Nausea: A feeling of sickness in the stomach that prompts the urge to vomit.

Nasogastric Tube (NGT): A tube placed through the nose into the stomach. It can be used to provide nutrition or can be used to provide relief due to ileus or obstructive symptoms.

Non-heme Iron: Iron found in plant-based foods such as grain, beans, fruits, vegetables, nuts, and seeds.

Oral Candidiasis (or Thrush): A fungal infection that causes white or red patches in the mouth and tongue, causing sore mouth, taste changes, or coated tongue. Thrush is common in adults with weakened immune systems because of medications or chemotherapy's side effects.

Oral Rehydration Solution: Type of drink made of water, glucose, sodium, potassium, and other electrolytes used to prevent and treat dehydration, particularly from diarrhea or vomiting.

Oral Supplement: A liquid or powder that provides additional calories, protein, vitamins, and minerals in the diet.

Oxaliplatin (Eloxitan®): An alkylating chemotherapy drug used to treat cancer, often used in combination with other chemotherapies.

Pancreas: Organ located in the abdomen that aids with digestion through production of enzymes and bicarbonate (exocrine function) in addition to producing hormones such as insulin and glucagon, which aid in blood glucose regulation (endocrine function).

Pancreatic Enzymes: The proteins made by the pancreas that aid in food digestion. The three types are amylase, lipase, and protease. Together these enzymes are commonly referred to as pancreatic juice.

Pancreatic Enzyme Replacement Therapy (PERT): Prescribed pancreatic enzymes taken at meals used to treat exocrine pancreatic insufficiency. These enzymes help mimic the function of a normal pancreas. Examples of prescription enzymes include Creon®, Pancreaze®, Pertzye®, Ultresa®, Viokace®, and ZenPep®.

Parenteral Nutrition: Nutrition or hydration provided intravenously (IV) into a vein bypassing the gastrointestinal tract.

Pemazyre® (Pemigatinib): Targeted therapy in the treatment of cholangiocarcinoma that binds to the fibroblast growth factor receptor (FGFR) found on the surface of the cancer cells to inhibit cancer growth.

Perihiliar Cholangiocarcinoma: Cancer originates in the bile duct's epithelial cells, just outside the liver.

Peripheral Line: A small, short plastic catheter placed through the skin into a vein to provide fluids, medications, or small amounts of nutrition.

Phosphorus: Mineral present in the body is a component of teeth, bones, and cell membranes involved in energy use and storage.

Phosphorus Additives: Compounds such as phosphoric acid, sodium phosphate, and sodium polyphosphate that is added to food to preserve moisture or color or enhance or stabilize the food.

Phosphorus Binders: Medications taken with meals that help prevent dietary phosphorus from being absorbed by the body.

Porcine: A scientific term used to describe a pig (pancreatic enzymes are derived from porcine).

Potassium: A mineral found in many foods that helps in heart function and muscle contraction.

Probiotic: Live microorganisms, the same or like those found in the gut, which may provide health benefits when consumed. These microorganisms are referred to as "good" or "friendly" bacteria that normally live in the digestive system without causing disease. They are found naturally in foods such as yogurt, kefir, or other fermented foods.

Protease: An enzyme secreted by the pancreas that breaks down proteins.

Protein: A nutrient found in foods such as meat, poultry, fish, eggs, peanut butter, nuts, dried beans, milk, cheese, yogurt, and soy products. The body uses proteins to build muscles and make natural hormones and steroids.

Radiation Therapy: Targeted doses of high-energy rays or particles used to kill cancer cells.

RELIZORB: A pancreatic enzyme cartridge containing lipase used for patients on continuous tube feedings.

Glossary

Resectable: Able to be treated with surgery.

Simethicone (Gas X® or Phazyme®): Medications used to remove excess gas in the intestinal tract by helping air in the stomach be more readily expelled by burping or passing gas. The drug does not prevent the accumulation of gas created by intestinal bacteria or from swallowed air or make intestinal gases dissolve.

Simple Sugars: Forms of sugar with little or no nutritional elements such as vitamins, minerals, protein, and fiber from the original plant products. Refined/simple carbohydrates include table sugar, brown sugar, raw sugar/turbinado, molasses, confectioners/powdered sugar, high fructose corn syrup, and honey. Concentrated refined/simple carbohydrates are found in desserts and sweet beverages.

Sodium: A naturally occurring mineral that aids in nerve and muscle function and helps to regulate fluid in the body.

Surgery: The removal, repair, or readjustment of organs and tissues, usually involving cutting into the body.

Survivorship: The focus on the health and well-being of a person with cancer from the time of diagnosis until the end of life. Includes the physical, mental, emotional, social, and financial effects of cancer that begin at the time of diagnosis and continue through treatment and beyond.

Tacrolimus (Prograf®): Immunosuppressive medication used after transplant to prevent organ rejection.

Targeted Therapy: A cancer treatment that uses drugs to target specific genes and proteins in cancer cells.

Torsemide (Demadex®): Diuretic medication used to increase water and salt excretion from the kidneys through urine.

Transplantation: A surgery to remove a diseased or injured organ and replace it with a healthy organ from another person, called a donor.

Unresectable: Not able to be treated with surgery.

Vitamin: A nutrient essential in small amounts to help the body's metabolic reactions occur properly.

Whipple Surgery: The surgical removal of the head of the pancreas, the lymph nodes near the head of the pancreas, the gallbladder, the duodenum (first part of the small intestine), and a small portion of the stomach called the pylorus.

Xerostomia: Abnormal mouth dryness that causes difficulty eating, talking, taste alterations, and/or thick ropy saliva.

Glossary

References

American Institute for Cancer Research

How to Prevent Cancer: 10 Recommendations

https://www.aicr.org/cancer-prevention/

New American Plate

Setting Your Table to Prevent Cancer

https://www.aicr.org/cancer-prevention/healthy-eating/
new-american-plate/

Malnutrition

White J, Guenter P, Jensen G, Malone A, Schofield M.
Consensus Statement: Academy of Nutrition and Dietetics
and American Society for Parenteral and Enteral Nutrition.
Journal of Parenteral and Enteral Nutrition. 2012;36(3):275-
283. doi:10.1177/0148607112440285

Cachexia

Fearon K, Strasser F, Anker S et al. Definition and
classification of cancer cachexia: an international
consensus. *The Lancet Oncology.* 2011;12(5):489-495.
doi:10.1016/s1470-2045(10)70218-7

Roeland E, Bohlke K, Baracos V et al. Management of
Cancer Cachexia: ASCO Guideline. *Journal of Clinical
Oncology.* 2020;38(21):2438-2453. doi:10.1200/
jco.20.00611

Nutrition After Duodenal Stent

- PANCAN UK Diet After a Stent or Bypass Surgery
  https://www.pancreaticcancer.org.uk/information/
  treatments-for-pancreatic-cancer/stents-and-
  bypass-surgery/diet-after-a-stent-or-bypass-
  surgery/

- PANCAN UK Eating After Duodenal Stent
  https://pancreaticcanceraction.org/wp-content/
  uploads/2017/11/PCA-BKLT-DuodenumStent-
  reprint-0316.pdf

- Ohio State University: Soft Diet After Gastrointestinal
  (GI Stent)
  https://healthsystem.osumc.edu/pteduc/docs/
  SoftDietAfterGastrointestinal(GI)Stent.pdf

References

Surgery Section

Cholecystectomy

- Nutrition Care Manual: Gallbladder Nutrition Therapy, Fat-Restricted Nutrition Therapy, Fat-Content of Food List
- Oncology Resource Toolkit: Low-Fat Diet
- Oncology Nutrition for Clinical Practice

Transplant

- Liver Transplant
  https://www.niddk.nih.gov/health-information/liver-disease/liver-transplant

- Diet and Transplantation
  https://www.kidney.org/atoz/content/nutritrans#

- Foods to Avoid After Transplant
  https://www.kidney.org/atoz/content/foods-avoid-after-transplantation

- Care After Kidney Transplant
  https://www.kidney.org/atoz/content/immunosuppression

- Liver Transplant for Cholangiocarcinoma Current Status and New Insights:
  https://www.ncbi.nlm.nih.gov/pmc/articles/PMC4598610/pdf/WJH-7-2396.pdf

- Current Status of Liver Transplantation for Cholangiocarcinoma:
  https://www.cancer.org/cancer/bile-duct-cancer/treating/surgery.html

- Nutrition Care Manual: Potassium Content of Food List
- NIDDK: Potassium: Tips for People with Chronic Kidney Disease
- National Kidney Foundation
  Guide to Low Potassium Diet Final 0.pdf

  https://www.kidney.org/atoz/content/potassium

Food Safety

- USDA Safe Food Handling and Preparation
  https://www.fsis.usda.gov/food-safety/safe-food-handling-and-preparation

- USDA Food Safety: A Need-to-Know Guide for Those at Risk
  https://www.foodsafety.gov/

Whipple

- Nutrition Care Manual: Whipple Surgery Nutrition Therapy
- Oncology Nutrition DPG: Diet After Whipple Surgery
  https://www.oncologynutrition.org/erfc/eating-well-when-unwell/diet-after-whipple-procedure

- Nutrition and Pancreaticoduodenectomy
  https://pubmed.ncbi.nlm.nih.gov/20581316/

- Nutrition Implications for Long-Term Survivors of Pancreatic Cancer Surgery
  https://aspenjournals.onlinelibrary.wiley.com/doi/abs/10.1177/0884533617722929

- Oncology Resource Toolkit: Malabsorption, Pancreatic Enzymes
- Oncology Nutrition For Clinical Practice

Nutrition Support

- Oncology in Clinical Practice
- RELiZORB
  https://www.relizorb.com/

Malabsorption

- Complete Resource Kit for Oncology Nutrition

Nutrition Management of Side Effects of Cancer Treatment

- Nutrition Care Manual
- Oncology Nutrition for Clinical Practice
- Frankly Speaking about Cancer. Eating Well During Cancer Treatment.
  https://www.cancersupportcommunity.org/sites/default/files/fsac/eating_well_for_cancer_survivors.pdf

- Eating Hints Before, During and After Cancer Treatment, National Cancer Institute
  https://www.cancer.gov/publications/patienteducation/eatinghints.pdf

- Nutrition for the Person with Cancer During Treatment, American Cancer Society.
  https://www.cancer.org/treatment/survivorship-during-and-after-treatment/staying-active/nutrition.html

- Iron Health Professional Fact Sheet.
  https://ods.od.nih.gov/factsheets/Iron-HealthProfessional/

Phosphorus Section

- Nutrition Care Manual: Phosphorus Content of Foods
- NIDDK: Phosphorus: Tips for People with Chronic Kidney Disease
  https://www.niddk.nih.gov/health-information/kidney-disease/chronic-kidney-disease-ckd/eating-nutrition

- National Kidney Foundation
  https://www.kidney.org/atoz/content/phosphorus

- Renal Dietitians DPG: Making Sense of Phosphorus

Resources Section:

https://www.cancer.org/treatment/caregivers/caregiver-resource-guide.html

NOTES

_____

_____

_____

_____

_____

_____

_____

_____

_____

_____

_____

_____

Patient
Support

A cholangiocarcinoma diagnosis can make you feel disconnected from your everyday life. This nutritional resource can strengthen your ability to deal with cancer by helping you to understand some basic principles of nutrition and offering you options that can best support you in your efforts.

The Cholangiocarcinoma Foundation (CCF) also offers an individualized mentoring program called CholangioConnect. Patients and caregivers are matched with survivors who can provide you with support and guidance throughout your cancer journey.

Additionally, you can find supportive educational materials on biomarker testing, clinical trials, and the patient registry on the CCF website.

You are invited to get more information about the free services and resources provided by the Cholangiocarcinoma Foundation by visiting cholangiocarcinoma.org.

Call toll free, Monday-Friday, 9 a.m. to 5 p.m.

Mountain Time, 1-888-936-6731, extension 8.

Email advocacy@cholangiocarcinoma.org

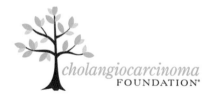

Nutrition
and
Cholangiocarcinoma

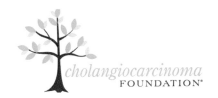

cholangiocarcinoma
FOUNDATION